2003

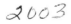
W9-ADS-749

ORGAN
TRANSPLANTS

ORGAN TRANSPLANTS

Other books in the At Issue series:

ORGAN TRANSPLANTS

James D. Torr, *Book Editor*

Daniel Leone, *President*
Bonnie Szumski, *Publisher*
Scott Barbour, *Managing Editor*

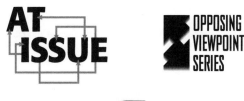

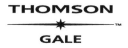

San Diego • Detroit • New York • San Francisco • Cleveland
New Haven, Conn. • Waterville, Maine • London • Munich

LIBRARY
UNIVERSITY OF ST. FRANCIS
JOLIET, ILLINOIS

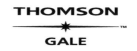

© 2003 by Greenhaven Press. Greenhaven Press is an imprint of The Gale Group, Inc., a division of Thomson Learning, Inc.

Greenhaven® and Thomson Learning™ are trademarks used herein under license.

For more information, contact
Greenhaven Press
27500 Drake Rd.
Farmington Hills, MI 48331-3535
Or you can visit our Internet site at http://www.gale.com

ALL RIGHTS RESERVED.
No part of this work covered by the copyright hereon may be reproduced or used in any form or by any means—graphic, electronic, or mechanical, including photocopying, recording, taping, Web distribution or information storage retrieval systems—without the written permission of the publisher.

Every effort has been made to trace the owners of copyrighted material.

LIBRARY OF CONGRESS CATALOGING-IN-PUBLICATION DATA

Organ transplants / James D. Torr, book editor.
   p. cm. — (At issue)
Includes bibliographical references and index.
ISBN 0-7377-1161-2 (pbk. : alk. paper) — ISBN 0-7377-1162-0 (lib. : alk. paper)
   1. Transplantation of organs, tissues, etc.—Moral and ethical aspects.
2. Medical ethics. I. Torr, James D., 1974– II. At issue (San Diego, Calif.)
RD120.7 .O737   2003
174'.25—dc21   2002067193

Printed in the United States of America

G
174,2
068

Contents

Introduction

"Despite continuing advances in medicine and technology, the demand for organs drastically outstrips the number of organ donors," states a United Network for Organ Sharing (UNOS) fact sheet. UNOS is a non-profit charitable organization that, under the authority of the federal government, maintains the United States' organ transplant waiting list and works to develop organ transplantation policies and raise awareness about organ donation. According to UNOS, the chronic shortage of organ donors is the most critical issue facing the field of organ transplantation. While 22,854 lifesaving organ transplant operations were performed in 2000, over fifty-eight hundred people died while waiting for a transplant—an average of more than fifteen every day. In February 2002, there were over seventy-nine thousand patients waiting for an organ transplant, up from less than fifty-five thousand in 1996.

Factors behind the organ shortage

Ironically, the increasing success rate of organ transplant procedures is one reason that organ transplant waiting lists have risen so dramatically since the late 1980s. The first organ transplants, performed in the late 1950s and 1960s, were characterized by high mortality rates; a major problem was that patients' immune systems often rejected the foreign organ. The introduction of the drug cyclosporine in the 1980s helped mitigate this problem, and organ transplants subsequently became less experimental and more routine. Statistics indicate that in 1998 organ transplant procedures were successful 70 to 95 percent of the time, depending on the organ being transplanted. With these increasing success rates, more doctors have recommended the procedures.

Another factor behind the organ shortage is that, according to UNOS, "relatively few deaths occur under circumstances that make [cadaveric] organ donation possible." There are two main types of organ donation: living-donor donation and cadaveric donation. Kidney transplants make up 95 percent of living-donor donations; the other 5 percent are largely from liver donations, a rare procedure in which an adult donates a portion of his or her liver to an infant. But the majority of kidney and liver donations, and virtually all pancreas, heart, and lung transplants, are removed surgically from donors shortly after their death. (By law, organs are only removed if the deceased carried an organ donor card or if family members give permission.)

Since the organs must be removed so quickly after death, cadaveric donors usually are individuals who have died in circumstances that make a swift determination of death possible: Among cadaveric donors in 1999, head trauma and cerebrovascular stroke accounted for 85 percent of all deaths. Thus, even if the number of people willing to donate organs increased at the same level as the demand for organ transplants, demand would outpace supply since only a minority of people die in circumstances that make cadaveric donation possible.

A final explanation for the organ shortage is Americans' general reluctance to become organ donors. In a 1993 Gallup poll, 85 percent of those surveyed said that they support organ donation, but only 37 percent said that they were "very likely" to donate their own organs, and 25 percent said they were "not at all likely." There are a variety of reasons that people may be uncomfortable with organ donation, but the Gallup poll zeroed in on a major one: 36 percent of respondents agreed that "thinking about your own death makes you uncomfortable." Organizations such as UNOS are dedicated to encouraging Americans to overcome this reluctance to become organ donors. To this end they often stress that organ donation is a lifesaving act, not one that should be associated with death.

Proposals to increase the number of organ donors

However, raising awareness about organ donation is a slow process, and the need for more organs is immediate. Thus the biggest dilemma facing the transplant community is, "How can the number of organs available for transplant be increased?"

One proposal is to reverse the current system in which doctors must obtain a patient's (or his or her family's) consent in order to remove organs after death. Under a policy of "presumed consent" all patients would be presumed to want to become organ donors unless they explicitly state otherwise. Presumed consent proposals have consistently been met with strong opposition, however, on the grounds that they violate an individual's right to make medical decisions for themselves.

"Mandated choice" or "required response" policies are less extreme alternatives to presumed consent. Advocates of mandated choice policies argue that rather than waiting for people to volunteer for organ donation, hospitals or government organizations should require individuals to state their preference about organ donation, perhaps when they obtain their driver's licenses or file tax returns. Texas, Colorado, and several other states have implemented required response policies, but, on average, rates of organ donation have not risen dramatically as a result.

One of the most controversial proposals is to provide individuals with some type of incentive to become organ donors. Such incentives could range from straight cash payments for living-donor organs to government assistance with funeral expenses for the families of cadaveric donors. Currently, proposals for compensated donation would likely be in violation of the 1984 National Organ Transplant Act, which makes it illegal to buy or sell human organs. Critics also charge that payment for organ donation could lead to a black market for human organs. In fact, such a black market already exists in India, where, according to a 1998 investigative report in the *New York Review of Books*, wealthy foreigners with end-stage renal disease pay thousands of dollars for human kidneys "donated" by impoverished Indians.

Given the ethical dilemmas surrounding proposals to increase organ donation, the medical community has searched for other ways to alleviate the organ shortage. Xenotransplantations, or cross-species transplantations, have been offered as one such solution. Surgeons transplanted a baboon heart into an infant nicknamed "Baby Fae" in 1982, but the child died three weeks later. More recently, pigs have been heralded as a potential source of organs. In January 2002, for example, scientists from the same laboratory that cloned Dolly the sheep in 1997 announced that they had genetically modified five piglets to make their organs more suitable for transplantation into humans.

Xenotransplantation raises a different set of ethical questions, however. Animal welfare activists have been very vocal in their opposition to xenotransplantation research. They also point to possible dangers associated with pig-to-human transplants. Xenozoonosis—the transmission of animal diseases to humans via blood or organ transplants—is a serious concern among scientists working on pig-to-human transplants. In 2000, the International Society for Heart and Lung Transplantation issued a report advising against further xenotransplantation until the virus risks are known, but the organization also concluded that "xenotransplantation has the potential to solve the problem of donor organ supply, and therefore research in this field should be actively encouraged and supported." Despite both the ethical and the epidemiological issues associated with xenotransplantation, the research holds promise for the thousands of patients on organ transplant waiting lists.

Researchers are also working on developing artificial organs. As of February 2002, five people have received fully self-contained artificial hearts. The artificial heart has rarely been used because it is still highly experimental and because recipients must be willing to have their own heart removed to make room for the artificial replacement. Although there are many technical hurdles to overcome in the field of artificial organs, researchers are hopeful: Various laboratories in the United States and around the world are developing artificial hearts, lungs, livers, pancreases, bladders, and blood.

In addition to developing artificial organs, scientists are working on techniques to grow human organs from a patient's own cells. Instead of waiting for a donor, for example, a patient in need of a heart transplant might one day only have to wait until researchers can grow one in the laboratory. Some of the research involved in tissue engineering is tied up with cloning and stem cell research, and thus raises ethical questions. Such research is also at the cutting edge of biotechnology, and therefore it may be decades before it bears fruit. Nevertheless, the medical community is eager to explore this potential solution to the organ shortage.

Alleviating the organ shortage

Although tissue engineering, artificial organs, and xenotransplantation provide hope for the future, the thousands of people currently on organ transplant waiting lists are counting on altruistic organ donation. As bioethicist Arthur Caplan explains,

> What is truly distinctive about transplantation is not technology but ethics. Transplantation is the only area in all of health care that cannot exist without the participation of the public. It is the individual citizen who while alive or af-

ter death makes organs and tissues available for transplantation. If there were no gifts of organs or tissues, transplantation would come to a grinding halt.

The field of organ transplantation is one of the miracles of modern medicine, but its power to save lives depends directly on the availability of organs. The authors in *At Issue: Organ Transplants* debate the various ways to increase the number of organs available for transplant and thus reduce the number of patients who die every day waiting for a new heart, liver, or kidney.

1

The United States Should Adopt a Policy of Presumed Consent Toward Organ Donation

Fady Moustarah

Fady Moustarah was a postgraduate student of general surgery at the McMaster University in Hamilton, Ontario, when he wrote this viewpoint for the 1997 Logie Medical Ethics Essay Contest.

Under the current system of organ donation in Canada and the United States, unless individuals expressly give their consent to donate organs, it is illegal for doctors to use their organs for transplant. In addition to costing thousands of lives each year, this policy is flawed because the majority of people support organ donation but simply fail to fill out organ donor cards. A system in which individuals were presumed to want to donate their organs after death—but could still choose not to by carrying a card or registering with the government—would save lives and better serve most people's wishes regarding organ donation.

Transplants involving cadaver organs are among contemporary medicine's greatest success stories because they mean an increased survival rate and better quality of life for people with end-stage organ failure (ESOF).

As well, "there is every expectation that [transplant results] will continue to improve in the future."[1] Unfortunately, demand for organs far outstrips supply and the rationing that results essentially condemns many patients to death. Medicine could, and should, move in a direction that would alleviate the need for these rationing decisions.

Saving life is a core moral principle in medicine; in fact, the principle of beneficence holds that physicians ought to find ways either to save the lives or to improve the quality of life of their ESOF patients. It is ethically unacceptable to ignore the plight of patients who could be saved.

From "Organ Procurement: Let's Presume Consent," by Fady Moustarah, *Canadian Medical Association Journal*, 1998. Copyright © 1998 by the Canadian Medical Association. Reprinted with permission.

13

Allocating life and death

How can we avoid allocation decisions and save the lives of those on transplantation waiting lists? Although several factors are involved, the major limiting factor in Canada is the inadequate supply of donor organs. This puts our line of attack in clear focus.

Canada currently has an opting-in policy, which means that organs are harvested only if someone has provided consent, and this system fails to meet the growing need. We must adopt a better procurement policy. In Alberta there have been suggestions to switch to an "opting-out" policy, a practice often referred to as "presumed consent." Although the idea has been floated within the transplantation field since 1968, it has not gained widespread support and governments have been reluctant to adopt it. Physicians might assume that this reluctance means the practice is morally objectionable, but they shouldn't be misled. A system of presumed consent not only will increase the organ supply but is also morally defensible because it better respects the individual autonomy that the current opting-in system strives so hard to protect.

Supply and demand

One author noted that "figures need not be invoked to remind us that we face a donor organ shortage."[2] Although I will rely on "figures," I will also emphasize that behind every one of them is a man, woman or child whose life is in jeopardy and can potentially be saved. In the US, for example, "there has been a 12.4% increase in the need for kidney, heart, liver, heart-lung and pancreas transplantation procedures between 1980 and 1990."[3] During this period the need for cadaver kidneys increased by 267%. In June 1991 more than 23,000 people were on the United Network for Organ Sharing waiting list—a 75% increase since 1987. Unfortunately, the supply of donor organs has remained relatively unchanged since 1980.

Canada is witnessing similar trends. Of the 1067 patients awaiting kidney transplantation in Alberta in 1990, only 551 underwent the procedure; among patients receiving dialysis in northern Alberta in 1992, half were on a transplant waiting list.

Our failure to seek an ethical alternative to the organ shortage passes a death sentence on many Canadians and a properly enforced system of presumed consent may help solve the problem. Studies from Belgium and Austria have shown that "the problem of chronic organ shortage can adequately be solved" with an opting-out system[4] and that there are "enough organ donors for all patients on the waiting list, at least for kidneys."[5] Thus, unless it can be proved that presumed consent is ethically unacceptable, we have a duty to pursue this option.

Autonomy and presumed consent

Respect for autonomy requires that we recognize that rational beings have inherent worth and their actions must result from their own deliberations. In Kantian terms, individuals should not be treated as means to an end because of their inherent value. From an ethical perspective, people should have authority over their own bodies; recognizing that saving the lives of ESOF patients is a desirable end does not by itself justify the removal of organs without prior consent. David Peters concluded that a person is considered to have "a legitimate and primary proprietary in his or her living or dead body" and thus "has first right to control what happens to his or her body before and after death."[6] So, how can we best realize the autonomous wishes of people concerning the disposition of their organs?

The [Canadian] Human Tissue and Gift Act (HTGA) of 1971 was adopted by all provinces to ensure that people had authority over their own bodies while also providing an opting-in system to encourage organ procurement. It states that cadaver organs can only be harvested if the donor has left explicit official consent, which is "binding and full authority for the . . . removal and use of the specified body parts." The only exception arises when a procurer "has actual knowledge of an objection thereto by . . . a person of the same or closer relationship to the person in respect of whom the consent was given."[7] In theory, the HTGA protects donor autonomy while presuming that only those who signed cards want to donate organs.

Such a presumption errs in its empiric foundation: most people who eagerly support organ donation and would also choose to receive a transplant have never signed their donor cards. Studies completed in Ontario and Alberta in 1985 showed that even though there was strong support for organ donation, "70% of individuals had not signed their donor cards." A 1992 study in Alberta found that 77% of respondents would like unlimited access to transplants yet "the percentage of unsigned donor cards has remained relatively constant."[8]

A system of presumed consent not only will increase the organ supply but is also morally defensible.

It appears that many people who support organ donation have difficulty envisioning their own deaths and find it hard to contemplate donating their organs, although other factors may be in play as well. If asked, many people who fail to sign donor cards would say that organ donation is desirable and noble. Therefore, we err when we assume that the absence of expressed consent implies a refusal to donate. Alternatively, *presuming* consent allows us to meet better the wishes of most people. Hence, presuming that the majority favour organ donation is the morally correct way to proceed because it finds its roots in the recognition of the *unexpressed* but autonomous will of most members of society.

I hesitate to say *unexpressed* autonomous will because with time a properly implemented policy of opting-out can effectively equate the failure to indicate refusal to donate with the indirect expression of consent. In other words, it would be safe to assume that people who have not registered an objection want to donate their organs. To avoid misinterpretation, massive amounts of public education would be needed before any shift to presumed consent. Debates and educational campaigns could be used to raise awareness of the need for organs, the success of transplants, medical criteria for death and the compatibility of organ donation and religious belief. In Singapore, where presumed consent has been the rule since 1987, all residents receive a letter upon attaining the age of majority. It states that they are presumed to consent to organ donation if they do not explicitly object to it; Muslims are considered objectors unless they opt in. For minors and mentally incompetent people, consent is sought from next of kin. With measures such as these, everyone should be able to make an informed decision.

Autonomy and next of kin

Besides failing to recognize the wishes of the majority, the current opting-in system violates individual autonomy on another level. Because of exceptions to the "consent is full authority" clause mentioned earlier, the HTGA means decisions are often made by relatives of the deceased. People who procure organs continue to seek permission from next of kin even though consent has already been given. This begs the question of whose rights and autonomy ought to be respected, those of the donor or those of the next of kin?

Presuming *consent allows us to meet better the wishes of most people.*

We make a huge moral mistake when we let the wishes of the next of kin take priority. Seeking such consent is also time consuming and often results in family distress when feelings of guilt and sorrow are prevalent. The time lost may result in tissue death and concomitant organ damage, and even lead to an objection to removal of an organ the deceased person had agreed to donate. The potential consequence is the loss of one more life.

Under our current system, there is little incentive for anyone to sign a donor card. As a potential donor I have to foresee my death, realize the need for organs and sign my donor card as a goodwill gesture, all the time realizing that my family's wishes might be given precedence over mine. The fact that these wishes often coincide is irrelevant. If I decide to object to organ donation and refrain from signing my card, my wishes may still be overlooked because families can give postmortem anatomical gifts upon request. It is difficult to distinguish between objectors and supporters of organ donation because even though no objectors sign their donor cards, not every person who fails to sign a card is an objector.

A policy of presumed consent can protect the wishes of objectors because their registered objections would not be subject to contravention. If they change their mind, the burden of cancelling their objection would be on them. As to those who choose not to object, a system of presumed consent allows for rapid removal of organs and meets the medical need for harvesting well-oxygenated tissue that improves the operation's success rate. By presuming consent, procurers would also be saving families unnecessary grief—they would no longer be asking questions at the worst possible time, questions that should not be asked in the first place.

Technical objections

Despite its appeal as an ethically acceptable method for procuring organs, a presumed-consent policy may face practical difficulties. However, solutions exist.

• Some say that an opting-out registry would become too complicated and would not be able to maintain uniformity across jurisdictional boundaries. This may have been true in the past, but technology and rapid communication mean that we can surely create a system to ensure that objectors can leave directives of their intentions, which would be readily available from a central registry. Also, objectors can still be protected even if we rely on the card system currently in use. Solutions are readily available in Austria, Belgium, Singapore and several other countries with presumed-consent legislation.

• Others argue that presumed consent will lead to distrust of the medical profession because physicians might confuse their role of saving the lives of potential donors with that of harvesting their organs, and may ease off on attempts to help a potential donor. This is simply an argument used by those who oppose the harvesting of organs. Today, procurement practices must meet stringent ethical criteria. This means that the life-saving team is kept separate from the organ-procuring team. The public needs to be informed of these safeguards, which will put unfounded fears to rest.

• Some fear that presumed consent means procurers might act too quickly in removing organs upon the declaration of death. This would be morally objectionable because it may harm members of the patient's family if they disagree with the medical criteria for death. If there is disagreement with the medical opinion physicians should respect that and give the family time to accept that the person is dead according to well-established and contemporary criteria.

Proponents of presumed consent need to show the public that they are not "organ vultures" but instead are trying to respect human freedom and dignity.

I can continue to list technical objections and technical solutions, but there is a way to resolve all such concerns. Presumed consent is designed to protect individual autonomy. Proponents of presumed consent need to show the public that they are not "organ vultures" but instead are trying to respect human freedom and dignity while trying to meet the increasing demand for organs.

The need for change

Altruistic voluntarism is not providing enough donor organs. Although most people appreciate the miracle of transplantation, many are reluctant to sign the donor cards that make the miracle possible. The opting-in policy currently in play fails to make enough organs available, fails to save the lives of some ESOF patients and fails to respect the autonomy of donors and nondonors alike. We need a radical change in policy that is both potentially effective and morally and socially desirable.

A presumed-consent policy can significantly increase the supply of organs while at the same time supporting the autonomous wishes of the majority concerning the use of body parts after death. Presumed consent would protect individual autonomy more than our current system, without being insensitive to the wishes of the next of kin. We will be making a great moral mistake if we fail to adopt an ethically acceptable policy of presumed consent that would help save many lives.

I will end by quoting David Longmore: "We either preserve the ancient laws that guarantee the inviolability of the dead, and the present rights of the next of kin, or we can rewrite those laws in favour of the living."[9]

Notes

1. Turcotte JG. Supply, demand and ethics of organ procurement: the medical perspective. *Transplant Proc* 1992;24(5):2140–2.

2. Guttmann RD, Guttmann A. Organ transplantation: duty reconsidered. *Transplant Proc* 1992;24(5):2179–80.

3. Evans RW. Need, demand and supply in organ transplantation. *Transplant Proc* 1992;24(5):2152–4.

4. Roels L, Vanrenterghem Y, Waer M, Christiaens MR, Gruwez J, Michielsen P. Three years of experience with a 'presumed consent' legislation in Belgium: its impact on multi-organ donation in comparison with other European countries. The Leuven Collaborative Group for Transplantation. *Transplant Proc* 1991;23(1Pt2):903–4.

5. Gnant MF, Wamser P, Goetzinger P, Sautner T, Steininger R, Muehlbacher F. The impact of the presumed consent law and a decentralized organ procurement system on organ donation: quadruplication in the number of organ donors. *Transplant Proc* 1991;23(5):2685–6.

6. Peter DA. Protecting autonomy in organ procurement procedures: some overlooked issues. *Milbank Q* 1986;64(2):241–70.

7. Cox M. *Human transplantation in Canada: the problems—the challenge.* Edmonton: Human Parts Banks of Canada; 1978.

8. Eley JA. *Organ procurement and transplantation: mandating appropriate legislation.* Edmonton: University of Alberta; 1992.

9. Kennedy I. The donation and transplantation of kidneys: Should the law be changed? *J Med Ethics* 1979;5:13–21.

The United States Should Not Adopt a Policy of Presumed Consent Toward Organ Donation

Troy R. Jensen

Troy R. Jensen won the 1999 James Baker Hughes Prize, a yearly award given for the best student-written paper on international economic law. The following viewpoint is excerpted from Jensen's winning paper.

Given the worldwide shortage of organs available for transplantation, some countries have adopted presumed consent laws under which doctors have the authority to remove recently deceased patients' organs unless the patient had registered as a non-donor. Brazil instituted such a law in 1998 but abolished the policy in the same year due to public opposition and reports of corruption and human rights violations. Other nations should also avoid presumed consent policies. Such policies are fundamentally at odds with an individual's right to control decisions regarding an invasion of his or her body.

Throughout the world, organ transplantation has emerged as an important medical advancement in solving the problem of end-stage organ failure. Over the years, the success rates of these transplants have significantly improved, providing the critically ill with a chance for a new life. . . .

Despite the advancements, the demand for organs significantly exceeds the available supply in countries around the world. This organ shortage is the most devastating obstacle that organ transplant patients face. As technology continues to expand, the number of patients diagnosed as potential organ transplant recipients increases. The disparity between supply and demand often leads to unethical and illegal methods of procuring needed organs. In many instances, the impoverished members of society supply organs for the privileged classes who can afford them. Poor people

Excerpted from "Organ Procurement: Various Legal Systems and Their Effectiveness," by Troy R. Jensen, *Houston Journal of International Law*, Spring 2000. Copyright © 2000 by the University of Texas at Houston. Reprinted with permission.

are often coerced to sell their kidneys through unethical and unsafe procedures for a meager fee. The organ deficit forces medical providers to decide which patients will receive life sustaining organs and which will not. Desperate patients purchase organs on the black market when they feel they can no longer afford to wait for an organ to be supplied through legal channels. . . .

Brazil's experience with presumed consent

The demand for organs overwhelmingly exceeds supply in the Brazilian organ market. In 1996, a mere 2.7% of Brazilians in need of transplanted organs received them. The low level of organ procurement in Brazil can be traced to both cultural and geographical factors. The human corpse is treated with particular reverence in Brazil and cremations are very rare. Many Brazilians are reluctant to consent to organ donation and many families are concerned with "desecrating" the remains of a loved one by allowing the harvest of organs. Furthermore, the long distances between remote rural towns and the rugged terrain in between impede the successful transportation of organs. Only 10% of the organs arriving at hospitals are in suitable condition for transplant. Rural hospitals lack the modern health care facilities and equipment necessary to perform these complex operations. Most transplants in Brazil are performed in Sao Paulo, where they average twenty-four per month in contrast to the U.S. average of fifty-five per day.

In response to this problematic organ deficit, Brazil decided to take legislative action to increase the supply of human organs for transplants. On January 1, 1998, Brazil enacted a law declaring all adults potential organ donors unless they filed for an exemption. The law allowed organ removal from the deceased without any notification or family consent. Upon death, if a person had not registered his or her intent not to be an organ donor with a special government agency, it was presumed that he or she had consented to donate his or her organs. The family of the deceased from whom organs were removed had no remedy under the law unless they could show that the deceased had filed for non-donor status. Furthermore, family members interfering with organ removal could have been sued. According to Federal Attorney Geraldo Brindeiro, the law allowed doctors to remove organs against the wishes of the family but did not legally obligate them to do so. Therefore, a doctor could have refused to remove organs if the family objected. In contrast, the legal coordinator for the health ministry warned that doctors who refused to extract organs, regardless of the family's wishes, could be prosecuted for failing to assist a person in need.

Despite the desperate need for human organs, scholars, the medical community, and the lay public expressed opposition to the Brazilian law. Critics feared the law would unfairly target the rural and uneducated who might not have realized that the new law made them potential organ donors. Others were concerned that the law might have led to the removal of organs from a non-donor even before his or her actual death due to conspiracy or mishandling of documents. A recent poll in Sao Paulo revealed that the law might actually have been counterproductive. While 75% of residents indicated a willingness to be an organ donor in 1995, this number fell to 63% in 1997 while the presumed consent law was being debated. The poll also found a significant drop in the willingness of residents to consent to donating the organs of deceased relatives.

The Brazilian Federal Medical Council, an independent association that monitors medical practices in the country, claimed that Brazil's infrastructure was incapable of administering such a complex plan. Some critics maintained that the problem was not a lack of voluntary donors, but rather a lack of structure capable of distributing organs safely and rapidly to hospitals across the country. Waldir Mesquita, president of the Federal Council of Medicine, believed the law violated "independence and freedom of belief," noting that millions of illiterate people could not afford to miss a day of work in order to pursue a non-organ donor identity card. Even groups of patients awaiting transplants openly opposed mandatory donations.

Presumed consent laws do not necessarily result in larger organ supplies.

The first patient to benefit from the presumed consent law was Jose Morais Reis, a fifty-five-year-old heart transplant recipient. Reis received the heart of an unidentified donor who was declared brain-dead minutes before the operation took place. According to Dr. Herbert Alves, Reis had been waiting four months for a donor heart and the transplant was a success. Despite this success story, hospitals worried that presumed consent would prompt a permanent backlash against organ donation by the people of Brazil who treat the human corpse with special reverence. The Federal Council of Medicine found fault with the requirement that two doctors, one being a neurologist, were required to determine whether a patient was legally dead. Council officials claimed this approach was unsophisticated, adding that it would be virtually impossible to find a neurologist to make that determination. However, some aspects of Brazil's law were embraced by medical professionals. One important feature of the law was the creation of a single waiting list for organ recipients. Before the law was passed, patients were placed on waiting lists at individual hospitals, and as organs became available, they were distributed to both private and public hospitals, via rotation. However, the lists at private hospitals where patients had more money, were considerably shorter than lists at public hospitals, which served the underprivileged. Doctors "admit to cases when patients have died in over-stretched emergency facilities at public hospitals, only for the body to be whisked away for a transplant operation to a well staffed private hospital, full of the modern machinery which might just have saved the patient's life."

Opposition to the law

Many Brazilians, fearing corruption and human rights violations such as the extraction of organs while the donor was still alive, rushed to register their non-donor status with the government. In Porto Alegre, 83% of the residents registered their refusal before the law officially took effect. Although it might appear that the people of Brazil overreacted to the presumed consent legislation, recent history suggests that their fears were not unfounded. Some residents, complaining of the disparity in health care between the rich and the poor, maintained their distrust in the government's ability to successfully run the program in a fair and just manner. In 1997, a well publicized account from rural Brazil informed citizens about a worker who awoke from a drunken stupor in the middle of a desolate field without his eyes. According to newspaper reports, his eyes had been removed surgically, yet the man was unable to remember anything about the experience. In July of 1997, Lucimaria Feitosa Santos went to the hospital due to chronic fatigue and high blood pressure. During the examination, doctors discovered that her right kidney was missing. Apparently, a Sao Paulo hospital had removed the kidney nine years earlier when Santos underwent investigative surgery for stomach pains. The Santos family is now suing the hospital for removing her kidney without consent.

The law was also attacked on the constitutional front with many critics claiming that it violated personal autonomy. When the law was first passed, the Federal Medical Council challenged the constitutionality of the law arguing that many people would not have the opportunity to oppose donation before their deaths. Federal Attorney Geraldo Brindeiro claimed that the law was constitutional but admitted that relatives of the deceased should have had a right to prevent the removal of organs for transplant. The Federal Medical Council appealed that decision to the Supreme Federal Tribunal in January 1998. According to its Federal Constitution, Brazil is a legal democratic state founded on the dignity of the human person. Article 3 of the document states that a fundamental objective of the Republic is to build a free, just, and solidary society and to reduce social and regional inequalities. The right to health is a social right guaranteed by the constitution. Perhaps the legislature was promoting this social right to health by ensuring that organs would be readily available to those in need. Although the government had the best intentions, public opinion and Brazil's medical organizations forced the government to abolish the presumed consent system. To bring the law in line with medical practice, Brazil now requires physicians to seek family authorization before harvesting organs.

Brazil is not the only country to adopt presumed consent laws. Until recently, most European countries were operating under presumed consent laws. Although in theory the law is very strict, enforcement of the law has been flexible. Most doctors choose to follow the wishes of family members even when the law would allow them to harvest organs without the consent of living relatives. European countries are beginning to turn to voluntary systems. For example, a treaty signed in Ovieda, Spain, in 1997 provides that the express and specific consent of a donor must be given before an organ is removed. The treaty prohibits the removal of organs from those unable to give consent.

Arguments for and against presumed consent

Presumed consent laws do not necessarily result in larger organ supplies. Although countries such as Austria, Belgium, France, and Spain have produced more organs than many countries that have voluntary donation systems, other countries such as Switzerland, Greece, and Italy actually have lower transplant rates than countries where organ donation is voluntary. Hong Kong legislators have consistently rejected presumed consent legislation and maintained a policy of requiring express consent since 1990. Although Hong Kong physicians originally agreed with the legislature, the Hong Kong Medical Association recently supported the adoption of a presumed consent system to address the urgent need for transplantable organs. With European countries abandoning the practice of presumed consent in favor of voluntary donation programs, it became more controversial for Brazil to maintain its presumed consent law. On the other hand, Singapore has administered a presumed consent system since 1987, and it has been successful in increasing the number of transplantable organs.

Presumed consent laws violate the principle that a person has a legal right to make decisions concerning an invasion of his body.

Advocates of presumed consent statutes claim they provide the most efficient method of maximizing organ procurement. In Austria, for example, the rate of cadaveric kidney procurement is double that of the United States and most European countries. Despite this success, the demand for organs significantly exceeds the supply even in countries with presumed consent laws. The problem in Brazil and other countries stems from incompetent administration and a lack of infrastructure rather than a defect in the law itself. Still, presumed consent countries are more successful at augmenting organ supplies than countries relying on altruism. According to one study, the success of presumed consent laws in other countries led 78% of transplant surgeons polled in the United States to favor the adoption of a presumed consent system.

Critics argue that despite success rates, presumed consent laws are constitutionally questionable because they violate personal autonomy. Specifically, opponents argue that presumed consent laws violate the principle that a person has a legal right to make decisions concerning an invasion of his body. Critics also cite the potential disparity between the rich and the poor. Many fear that the underprivileged will be less likely to exercise autonomy, especially since most are illiterate and legally disenfranchised. Others are concerned that altruism and charity will lessen in the face of such laws. Critics also worry that organs will be harvested from people who have registered as non-donors due to administrative deficiencies. Others worry that anxious physicians will extract organs before a donor is truly brain-dead.

Many arguments have been advanced to counter these criticisms. Those in favor of presumed consent argue that because organ donation is generally supported and potential donors are given the opportunity to opt-out, individual liberty is not significantly hampered. Proponents further argue that the slight inconvenience of registering actually promotes individual freedom by expressly ensuring that a donor's desires are carried out, rather than leaving the decision to the family. Supporters of presumed consent also contend that a person can experience altruism by simply deciding not to opt-out of the donation system.

Another advantage of a presumed consent system is that it is easier to manage than voluntary consent. For example, if there is no registered objection to organ donation, a transplant surgeon can remove organs without contacting the next of kin for consent. By reducing the lapse of time between death and organ extraction, there is a better chance that the transplant will be successful because the organ will be fresher. However, logic would suggest that a database indicating consent to organ removal would be as equally timesaving as a database indicating non-consent. Proponents of presumed consent point out that a properly functioning presumed consent system provides important spillover benefits. Not only will the transplant rate increase, but the success rate will increase also. As the pool of available organs increases, a physician will be better able to implant an organ with tissue matching that of the donee. An increased supply also eliminates the temptation to obtain organs through unethical means such as the black market. This in turn will diminish underground kidnapping rings that currently affect countries across Latin America. A presumed consent system would also positively affect taxpayers by reducing the amount of government spending on dialysis treatment for patients awaiting kidney transplants. . . .

Compulsory donation is indeed an oxymoron.

In October 1998, the Brazilian government abolished its presumed consent law. With opposition from the Brazilian Medical Association and the Federal Council of Medicine, as well as the general public, the law was destined to fail. Furthermore, the law was ineffective because most doctors were unwilling to harvest organs against the wishes of family members, even though the law required them to do so. The reaction of panicked citizens who rushed to public offices to register themselves as non-donors also weakened the effectiveness of the law. Not only did the law fail due to opposition, it was also impractical. The lack of infrastructure needed to maintain the intended register of recipients, as well as the inability to transport organs efficiently, further led to the law's demise.

Presumed consent, which has been replaced by voluntary systems in most European countries, is a quickly dissipating method of organ procurement. Compulsory donation is indeed an oxymoron. Although the organ supply might be augmented by such a system, particularly when education programs or conscription are instituted, the system is undesirable due to its infringement on personal autonomy and liberty.

3

A Policy of Mandated Choice Would Be Better than One of Presumed Consent

Dustin Ballard

At the time this viewpoint was written, Dustin Ballard was a medical student at the University of Pennsylvania.

A policy of presumed consent—which mandates that individuals must opt out of donating their organs—is ethically problematic. Such a policy would create the possibility that doctors would violate people's bodies without their consent. A better system would be to require individuals to make an explicit choice about organ donations—perhaps when they apply for their driver's licenses or file their taxes. Such a policy would likely increase levels of organ donation while also ensuring that an individual's choices regarding organ donation are respected.

When John Doe obtained a fake ID he may have anticipated difficulties with the law, but he probably never dreamed of the actual consternation that his piece of plastic could cause. In this week's episode of *ER*, young John Doe, injured in a motor vehicle accident, arrives in the Emergency Department in critical condition. Subsequent resuscitation efforts are unsuccessful and, after identifying an organ donor sticker on Doe's fake driver's license, the ER staff begins procedures to harvest his organs. They soon realize, however, that the ID picture does not match the victim. And now they have no idea who this man is or how old he is and have no way of getting in touch with his family. Given these facts, and the quickly moving stopwatch of transplant organ viability, they are faced with a difficult decision—should they take John's organs for transplant without any indication of his consent?

If John lived in Belgium, this question would be answered without a second thought. Belgium and a number of European and South American

From "To Take Without Permission? Presumed Consent for Organ Harvest in the ER," by Dustin Ballard, *Bioethics on NBC's* ER, March 23, 2000. Copyright © 2002 by The American Journal of Bioethics and Bioethics.net. Reprinted with permission.

LIBRARY
UNIVERSITY OF ST. FRANCIS
JOLIET, ILLINOIS

countries have attempted to address the shortage of transplant organs by instituting a policy that is often referred to in the literature as "presumed consent." Under the Belgian construct, the state makes the assumption that people are willing donors of organs after death, unless they explicitly "opt-out." The policy has been hailed by many as an unqualified success—after 10 years, less than 2% of the Belgian population "opts-out" and their organ-donation rate is one of the highest in the world.

So, in Belgium, this scenario wouldn't cause much confusion, but *ER* is not set in Belgium, and the US does not have a "presumed consent" organ harvest policy. Instead, the US operates on an "explicit consent" system under the Uniform Anatomical Gift Act that "gives all competent adults legal authority to decide for themselves whether or not they wish to become organ donors after death." Given the recent high profile case of Walter Payton* and the country's increasing organ deficit, however, there are many that are beginning to insist that the US adopt a policy similar to Belgium's. As of November 1999, there were 66,500 patients on organ waiting lists in the United States and it is estimated that 4000 of them will not receive an organ before dying. The number of patients in need of transplant has skyrocketed 212% over the past 12 years, primarily due to the increased incidence of Hepatitis C, and while organ donation rates have increased as well, they've only done so at a rate of 52%—just one-quarter of current need. Yet the pool of potential donors remains undertapped. For example, last year there were 15,000 patients with fatal head injuries in the United States—all of whom were potential organ donors but out of those 15,000, only 5400 actually became donors.

A policy of mandated choice or "required response" would require that all competent individuals make an explicit choice about organ donation.

Thus, while some may object to aspects of priority criteria for waiting lists and paradigms for distribution, the solution to the organ-shortage problem seems straightforward. If we were to institute a national policy of "presumed consent" we could significantly alleviate the nation's organ distribution headache. But wait; let's not get carried away, things are not that simple. . . .

A policy of presumed consent is ethically problematic regardless of its potential benefit for several reasons. First, the use of the term in relation to organ harvesting is somewhat disingenuous. "Presumed consent" presumes that "it is legitimate to take organs without explicit consent because those from whom the organs are taken would have agreed had they been asked when they were competent to respond."[1] The trouble with this presumption, at least in this country, is that on a case-by-case, it is not necessarily true. A 1993 Gallup Poll found that 69% of Americans would be "very likely" or "somewhat likely" to grant formal permission to have their organs harvested after death. Even counting the "somewhat

---

*NFL running back Walter Payton announced in February 1999 that he needed a liver transplant. Payton did not receive one and died that November.

likely" population, this still leaves over 30% of Americans who would not agree with a "presumed consent" policy for themselves. This can be contrasted with the other common use of the "presumed consent" concept—in the emergent treatment of incompetent patients in the Emergency Room—where there is near unanimous approval of unauthorized life-saving interventions. The Belgian system attempts to answer this criticism by allowing for an "opt-out." An "opt-out" system allows people, who, for religious or other reasons, wish that their body be "respected" after death, to withdraw themselves from presumed consent. This exception to the rule is problematic, though, if these people are not aware of the process or do not understand it completely. The burden of ensuring the respect for their preferences has been shifted on to them rather than on the state, and the association of organ transplantation with "donation" and "gifting" has been demeaned. This movement away from both altruism and autonomy is troubling.

Another, related, difficulty with presumed consent is that its use in a non-emergent situation sets a precedent that has the potential to erode the utility of the notion of informed consent. In their excellent sociological exploration of the phenomenon of organ transplantation, *Spare Parts,* Renee Fox and Janet Swazey offer a relevant warning about its dangerous momentum: "We have come to believe that the missionary-like ardor about organ replacement that now exists, the overidealization of the quality and duration of life that can ensue, and the seemingly limitless attempts to procure and implant organs that are currently taking place have gotten out of hand."

Fox and Swazey would have us ask whether it is worth it to trade a weakening in the concept of informed consent in order to transiently increase the organ donor pool. If we are willing to make this trade then what future utilitarian tradeoffs will we be willing to make if the organ deficit continues to grow? How much resolve will we have in protecting ethical principles of informed consent and patient autonomy?

A better policy

So, where are we left? Well, we have gained a further measure of appreciation for the dilemma that the ER staff face tonight. Violating a person's body, even when it is no longer alive, without consent, is clearly a dangerous precedent to set. At the same time, a significant majority of people, when polled, say they are willing to donate their organs after death—and it is a travesty to waste those organs. I believe that what is needed is a middle ground between our current system and presumed consent—one such as mandated choice.

A policy of mandated choice or "required response" would require that all competent individuals make an explicit choice about organ donation and protects this choice from any sort of familial veto. This process could be completed at a number of possible venues—prior to applying for a driver's license, on their tax form, or at the post office. This approach has several advantages: it removes the barrier of familial veto, requires people to consider organ donation in a more relaxed setting, and increases public awareness of the organ shortage and putatively organ donation rates without unduly jeopardizing individual autonomy. Of course, the process of implementing mandated choice would be delicate and it would have to be complemented by a comprehensive but non-coercive education campaign to educate the public not only about the organ shortage, but also the life expectancy and quality of life of organ recipients.

So, back to the dilemma in the ER. Mandated choice only obliquely helps us with this situation. It does so in that if we rely on its preservation of the principle of consent we are required to advise the ER staff to abandon attempts to harvest John Doe's organs—unless, of course, they could find proof of his real identity.

Note

1. Veatch RM, Pitt SB. The myth of presumed consent: ethical problems in new organ procurement. Caplan AL, Coelho D, editors. The ethics of organ transplants: the current debate. Amherst, NY. Prometheus Books: 1998:147.

4

Raising Awareness About Organ Donation Is Better than Presumed Consent or Mandated Choice

Phil H. Berry Jr.

Phil H. Berry Jr. is a practicing physician and served as president of the Texas Medical Association from 1997 to 1998.

The organ shortage in the United States, which leads to the deaths of thousands of people each year, could be eradicated if Americans would overcome their reluctance to become organ donors. Polls indicate that a majority of Americans are willing to become organ donors, yet relatively few actually do so. Proposals to "presume consent" for organ donation violate individual rights, and mandated choice systems—such as those in which individuals must decide about organ donation when they get their driver's licenses—force people to make an important choice in an uninformed and rushed manner. The most effective way to increase organ donation is to raise public awareness about it—families that discuss the issue are much more likely to permit a loved one's organs to be donated after death.

Perhaps no field of medicine is as exciting or is packed with so much emotion as the field of transplant medicine. With the advent of cyclosporine as an anti-rejection medication in 1980, the success rate of transplantation skyrocketed, promising the "gift of life" to many who heretofore were faced with certain death. I experienced firsthand the roller coaster of emotions as the hepatitis B virus I contracted in the operating room slowly destroyed my liver over the span of 3½ years. After two episodes of hepatic coma, punctuated by gastrointestinal bleeding from varices, I was placed on the waiting list for a liver transplant at Baylor University Medical Center in Dallas. Though I realized that a tragedy

Excerpted from "Ethics in Transplantation," by Phil H. Berry Jr., *Texas Medicine,* February 1997. Copyright © 1997 by the Texas Medical Association. Reprinted with permission.

must occur in someone else's life for me to have a chance, I was not too concerned at that time about ethics in this process.

Now I have the luxury of retrospectively considering the ethical concerns many people have addressed and continue to address to bring order to a system that is so important to so many people. [As of 1997] some 47,000 patients are on the waiting list awaiting organs and about 3000 will die each year because of the scarcity of organs in our country. . . .

Just as smallpox was eradicated from the face of the earth as a medical problem, we could have the same effect for those 47,000 people on the waiting list if we had enough organs donated for transplantation. Basically, the American public needs a major attitude adjustment. Some 3000 people die annually while waiting for an organ. I shudder when I think of that desperate feeling of wondering if I would even have a *chance* to survive, realizing that a tragedy must occur in someone else's life for me to survive.

Four proposals to increase organ donation

Many solutions to the problem have been suggested. The most current and viable are presented here.

Presumed consent

In three European countries (Austria, Belgium, and France), organ procurement legislation is based on the principle of *presumed consent*. In this situation, everyone is presumed to be an organ donor at death unless he or she opts out in advance. This system has satisfied the demand for organs in these countries, and the waiting lists are not increasing. Why hasn't this method been accepted more widely? The Council of Europe in 1978 recommended presumed consent legislation for the continent, but only these three countries are currently using this method. The rejection appears to be based on the apparent violation of individual choice, dignity, and autonomy. Some feel that altruism is inhibited also. Certainly in our legal climate in the United States, presumed consent would be subject to violations of individual rights at every turn.

The American public needs a major attitude adjustment.

This concept appeals to me, however, and might really be worth all the work it would take to change the attitude of most of the American public. For presumed consent to work, an effective and almost foolproof mechanism to document an individual's decision to opt out would be essential. The role of the family in the decision process would be minimized, and the need to address this issue at a stressful time would be obviated. Many proponents of presumed consent feel that it *enhances* the autonomy of the individual serving as the source of the organs. However, the UNOS [United Network for Organ Sharing] Subcommittee on Presumed Consent concluded in June 1993 that this model offers inadequate safeguards for the protection of individual autonomy of prospective donors and should not be part of any reform of the organ donation process. Instead, the subcommittee recommended the policy of "required response."

Mandated choice

With the concept of *mandated choice*, individuals would decide at a predetermined time (possibly at the renewal of a driver's license or some other state-mandated task) to be or not be an organ donor. In other words, they would be given the opportunity to make a choice, either positive or negative, and this choice would be made public knowledge. By requiring people to make a decision and contemplate their own death as well as the disposition of their bodies after death, a major obstacle would ostensibly have to be addressed and confronted. Many consider the reluctance to do this one of the main reasons organs are not donated.

Perhaps mandated choice would protect, and even enhance, individual autonomy. Families would have knowledge of the deceased relative's wish in this regard and would be more at ease with the process of donation. The downside of mandated choice is, of course, the "no" decision that might be registered, which becomes a huge roadblock for a family at the time of death. Dr Aaron Spital prompted a Gallup poll study that indicated 82% of the respondents believe the best approach to organ donation is for each adult to decide the issue for himself or herself. Only 14% felt family members should make this decision, showing tremendous support for self-determination. Another aspect of this study revealed that 76% of respondents *who had given this issue a great deal of thought* would be willing to donate, as opposed to 20% of those who had not. Of the 30% who had decided previously to donate, 95% would do so under a mandated choice plan; furthermore, of the 58% who had been undecided previously, 56% would do so under mandated choice. This does appear to be an acceptable method of increasing organ donation, and in 1994 was endorsed by UNOS and by the CEJA [Council on Ethics and Judicial Affairs] at the interim meeting of the AMA [American Medical Association] in 1993.

Required request

In this circumstance, hospital personnel (physicians, nurses, and others) or organ procurement personnel would be required to ask families whether or not they would consider donating their loved one's organs when death occurs. The decedent's wishes may or may not be known to the family and families may resent this request at such a sensitive time. As a result, requests many times are not made so as not to hurt the family's feelings or for fear of rejection.

Preferred status

The concept of preferred status rewards organ donors with a modest but definite recognition for their willingness to participate in the system, similar to crediting blood donors if they need blood in the future. Points, or some other value, would be given that would make it somewhat easier for that individual to receive an organ, if necessary, in the future. Obviously, a significant degree of public education would be involved.

From theory to practice

The good news according to a 1993 Gallup poll is that 95% of Americans are aware of transplantation and as many as 75% say they would be willing to donate an organ at their death. The bad news is that the Texas experience in asking people to make a choice at the time of driver's license renewal ranged from a 3% positive response 2 years ago to a high of 20% positive last year, when it was realized that the Department of Public Safety (DPS) computers were defaulting to "no" on the license. Although this was subsequently corrected, these numbers still do not match up with the Gallup poll numbers. An encouraging 60% positive response has been recorded in Colorado on driver's license renewals with mandated choice, but this is the only state with numbers this good.

In our legal climate in the United States, presumed consent would be subject to violations of individual rights at every turn.

As chairman of the legislative committee on organ donation appointed by Representative Ron Lewis (D-Mauriceville), I have had a wonderful opportunity to influence the formulation of Texas law, and our transplant laws have some unique features. At present, we do request a choice at the time of driver's license renewal, and a positive response by persons older than 18 years will insure their organs being donated (individual autonomy), even against their families' wishes. The state of Illinois has been innovative about public awareness and has two mailings before the driver's license renewal is sent, which appeal clearly to the altruistic spirit of people and outline the advantages of organ donation before the driver appears in a renewal line. When asked whether or not the individual wants to be a donor, only a "yes" answer is recorded and any negative responses are discarded. Letters from the Secretary of State and other state officials accompany the first two mailings, thus attaching themselves to a "mom and apple pie" cause and making some political hay. Whatever, the positive responses to this system hover consistently from 30% to 35%!

If approximately 75% of the American public expresses willingness to donate an organ after death (Gallup), this overwhelming public support, coupled with the low number of procured organs, led to the conclusion by public policy analysts that the low procurement rate results from the failure of health care providers to request donation from families of donor-eligible patients. An excellent study (required request) was developed to look comprehensively at just how organ, tissue, and cornea procurement works in actual clinical practice. Twenty-three hospitals in Pittsburgh and Minneapolis–St Paul participated in the study to determine such factors as the ability of health care professionals to identify donor-eligible patients, the frequency with which health care professionals approach families about donation, rates of consent to donation by families, and the factors associated with successful procurement. Almost 19% of organ-eligible cases were patients older than 59 years, and 98% died in the intensive care unit. Of the 170 organ-eligible cases for which donation was requested and a decision known, only 46.5% donated. Families of younger patients were more likely to donate than those of older patients. When a physician or nurse (clinician) was involved in the requesting process, consent was about 51% as opposed to 66% when a social worker or member of the clergy was involved. Health care professionals with training in requesting organs were more likely to ask for the organ but were no more successful than those with no formal training. This study raises some questions about the two central assumptions of US public policy on organ donation: that health care professionals fail to ask families for organs, and that, if asked, families will donate. The findings of this study suggest that any attempt to increase organ donation must address the families' reluctance.

The downside of *mandated choice* is that it artificially forces people to choose what they want done at some time in the future. A common fear, particularly among minorities, is that those willing to donate may be declared dead too soon. This fear is likely to be compounded by asking people to make their decision in an uninformed and rushed manner, eg, standing in a crowded line renewing a license on your lunch hour and being late to return to work. Indeed, our own Texas experience indicated a 97% "no" response when we started requested choice 3 years ago. Granted this was because the computers were set to a "no" default if someone was undecided, but even by correcting the problem last year, the positive response has only risen to about 20%. I remain convinced that more altruism exists in Texas than is manifest by the driver's license experience, and perhaps we should heed the wisdom of our Illinois peers. Strong consideration (as indeed suggested by many Texas transplant workers) must be given also to simply dropping the required request by DPS officials to prevent "no" from showing up on the driver's license. In the emergency room or intensive care unit when the discussion of organ transplantation arises and a "no" appears on the license, the experience of medical personnel indicates a virtual impossibility in convincing the family to donate their loved one's organs.

Changing attitudes

What really counts in our present-day society? Every study done has shown that *the single biggest factor in whether organs are donated is whether this issue was discussed in the family environment before the death of a loved one occurs.* The family's knowledge of the patient's previous wishes is central to deciding whether or not to donate!! When a bleeding cerebral aneurysm struck down a 30-year-old housewife in Brazoria, Texas, on October 26, 1986, her husband donated her liver for me—the gift of life—because they had discussed organ donation before she died. We can talk about required request, mandated choice, presumed consent, and a host of theoretical solutions, but I am convinced that until family members communicate with each other and realize what this gift of life can do for others, we will not begin to make any headway in relieving the burden for those 47,000 people waiting for their second chance. This problem can and will be solved by a change of attitude in our country. It will not be easy, but it can be done.

On March 3, 1996, I had the unique opportunity to address the congregation of the First Baptist Church of Brazoria, the home church of my donor and her family. Being able to stand before them and publicly thank them for the love given to me, the gift of life, gave them a sense of closure as they expressed how happy they were that I was doing so well and that part of her was still alive and continuing to help others. Is that not what organ donation is all about?

5

Compensating People for Organ Donation Could Alleviate the Organ Shortage

Gregory E. Pence

Gregory E. Pence is a professor of philosophy at the University of Alabama at Birmingham and the author of Re-Creating Medicine: Ethical Issues at the Frontier of Medicine *and* Classic Cases in Medical Ethics.

Under a 1984 federal law, it is illegal for hospitals, or anyone else, to offer financial incentives to people to donate their organs. This law is intended to safeguard medical ethics, but it is actually unethical for the medical community to ignore approaches that could alleviate the current organ shortage. Compensation for organ donation need not mean the unrestricted sale of human body parts. Instead, the government could implement a well-regulated system in which living donors receive payment for a kidney or other nonvital organ. Also, the families of posthumous organ donors could receive some type of compensation. At the very least the government should experiment with such incentives on a limited scale, to test their effectiveness.

> *He who saves a fellow creature from drowning does what is morally right, whether his motive be duty or the hope of being paid for his trouble.*
> —John Stuart Mill, *Utilitarianism*

In February 1999, famous NFL running back Walter Payton announced that he needed a liver transplant; he didn't get one and died that November. In 1997, more than 1,130 Americans died while waiting for a matching liver. Yet there is a way to increase the donation of livers that we have never tried.

Physicians in 1954 witnessed the first kidney transplant at the Peter Bent Brigham Hospital in Boston, and since then, the demand for donated kidneys has far surpassed the supply. In 1967, Christiaan Barnard

Excerpted from *Re-Creating Medicine: Ethical Issues at the Frontier of Medicine,* by Gregory E. Pence (Boston, MA: Rowman & Littlefield, 2000). Copyright © 2000 by Rowman & Littlefield Publishers, Inc. All rights reserved. Reprinted with permission.

performed the first heart transplant in Cape Town, South Africa. In 1976, discovery of the antirejection drug cyclosporin A enabled some transplant recipients to live for decades. Years later, livers and lungs were also successfully transplanted. These surgical achievements caused the demand for organs to grow exponentially.

We might just be able to push up the supply of organs with only modest use of monetary incentives.

One of the great taboos in transplant medicine has been against the rational discussion of using financial incentives to increase the donation of organs for these life-saving transplants. Almost universally, transplant surgeons condemn this option. Some U.S. bioethicists have followed suit, claiming that "rewarded giving" is unethical.

I believe that it's time for financial incentives to be carefully considered. . . .

To say that we need to think about using money to increase the supply of organs does not mean that we need to abruptly move from an altruistic, voluntary system to a crass, "anything goes" commercial system. Ethics is about drawing lines, and we might just be able to push up the supply of organs with only modest use of monetary incentives.

Three general methods using monetary incentives could increase organ transfers. The first, and most controversial, is a *pure market system,* a system that could work only for kidneys, bone marrow, and possibly lobes of regenerable livers. This system would allow a competent adult to sell, for example, one of his kidneys to another person on an open market, where buyer and seller negotiate the price. The second is a *regulated system* where a mediating agency sets a uniform price and guarantees conditions on both sides, such as the informed consent of the seller and, for the buyer, the quality of the organ bought. The regulating agency could also pay the cost of acquiring the organ, so that wealth does not affect who receives the organ. The final system is *rewarded cadaveric donation,* which consists of paying families to encourage them to donate organs of brain-dead relatives (also known in medicine as "cadaveric donations"). . . .

Background: reimbursing for human organs

Obviously, the possible exchange of money in organ transfers creates a lot of moral concern, and because every moral issue has a pedigree, the history of this concern is enlightening.

Sometimes in U.S. medicine, the public first hears about a good idea under the worst of circumstances, for example, when an idea is first espoused by a famous eccentric. Such death by association came when Jack Kevorkian publicly supported physician-assisted dying ("Kevorking" the issue) and when Chicago physicist Richard Seed announced he wanted to clone himself ("Seeding" the issue).

The earliest blow to the rational consideration of paid organ donation may have come from the controversial origins in the United States of paid *blood* donation, a system begun by a similar eccentric. Francis H. Bass, a former used-car salesman, started the first commercial blood bank in 1955 as a way to make a lot of money for himself. His blood bank battled non-profit, hospital-based blood banks, which took the moral high road that all donation of blood should be unpaid. The hospitals refused to do business with Bass, but he sued them and won when the Federal Trade Commission ruled in 1964 that the hospitals were in violation of free trade.

Nevertheless, the idea of paying for blood never transcended its eccentric origins. Had a distinguished physician and a proper hospital proposed to pay for blood, things might have been different.

The fatal blow to paid organ donation came from another person in this undistinguished line, businessman H. Barry Jacobs of Virginia. In 1983, Jacobs announced plans to start International Kidney Exchange, Ltd., an organization through which competent adults could buy and sell kidneys. The abhorrent part was that he planned on using indigent immigrants as sources for his organs.

What is the strongest argument for rewarded organ donation? . . . It's quite simple: doing so would save many lives.

At the time, such a business was not illegal in Virginia or in the United States, and Jacobs announced that his brokerage fees would make his operation "a very lucrative business." Jacobs's proposed business, and the way he talked about it, painted a morally repugnant picture: affluent people buying the kidneys of desperately poor people recently arrived in the United States, with unscrupulous brokers pocketing huge fees.

In reaction, a House subcommittee chaired by Albert Gore held hearings and recommended criminalizing the sale of organs; Congress soon followed its recommendation. Monetary incentives for organ donation became illegal, a violation of federal law, under the National Organ Transplantation Act of 1984, punishable by ten years in prison and a $500 thousand fine.

The 1971 publication of Richard Titmuss's *The Gift Relationship: From Human Blood to Social Policy* had previously dealt another blow to the impartial discussion of financial incentives for organ donation. Titmuss, an English sociology professor, disliked many aspects of American life. Parts of his 1968 book, *Commitment to Welfare,* spelled out this scorn with a vengeance. This book lambasted the U.S. medical system, which Titmuss saw as evil compared with the good, free, National Health Service, which—at least in theory and in those good old days—provided free, equal medical coverage for all English citizens.

Titmuss could not understand how any system with financial incentives and co-payments could be good, nor could he envisage the English system ever being inferior to the American system. In Titmuss's opinion, desires for profits corrupted the U.S. medical system, and U.S. physicians made obscene incomes, especially the overabundant specialists. . . .

So it was no surprise that his follow-up book, *The Gift Relationship,* expressed the same scorn and was meant to be a reductio ad absurdum of the American way of collecting blood. As Titmuss painted it, the contrast seemed stark and obvious: Americans bought blood from money-seeking alcoholics and prisoners, both of whom often carried blood-borne diseases and who were motivated to lie. In contrast, the altruistic English lined up good-naturedly and rolled up their sleeves for the needy. English blood was pure and free; American blood was dirty and bought. Need one say there was symbolism here?

As Douglas Starr observes in his masterful book on the history of blood, "Titmuss's book hit a public nerve. It generated scores of reviews in the news media and scholarly journals. It created a ripple effect. . . . The public now saw [as sources of American blood] the derelict and the prisoner."

Titmuss's book conveyed the residual impression that Americans had erred by allowing blood to be commercialized. Given such an impression, it was unlikely that organ donation ever had any real chance of being similarly commercialized. There was a big battle here between good and evil. We had messed up once by choosing evil, and we certainly shouldn't choose that side again.

Alas, Titmuss never revealed the fact that the English never got enough blood through altruistic donation and had to buy blood from the United States. The English learned this painful fact in the 1980s, after imported American blood infected many surgical patients there with HIV infections. . . .

Arguments for rewarded donation: saving lives

What is the strongest argument for rewarded organ donation? The answer is a direct one, appealing to life itself and not simply to indirect benefits. It's quite simple: doing so would save many lives. More than three thousand Americans die each year while waiting for an organ transplant that never occurs. But it's not clear that this has to happen.

At this moment, more than eleven thousand Americans are becoming jaundiced while waiting for a donated liver. Every year since 1998, one thousand of these people have died. Another four thousand Americans are turning ash-gray from failing circulation, as they wait for a heart. During the 1990s, 750 or more people died each year awaiting a heart transplant. By the end of 2000, more than forty thousand Americans will have died since 1988 awaiting an organ transplant.

So year after year, thousands of people die unnecessarily. Medicine has the scientific capacity, the facilities, and the personnel to save them, but the taboo against rewarded donation prevents it from doing so.

Isn't it . . . hypocritical that the only people not *paid in the whole system of organ transplantation are the families of the donors?*

In reviewing past discussions of paid organ transfer, I am struck by the fact that no one on either side emphasizes the huge numbers of lives lost as a result of not permitting financial incentives for organ donation. Indeed, this loss is sometimes treated by opponents of financial incentives as almost mundane, as if it should be obvious that thousands of lives *must* be sacrificed on the altar of a non-coarsened social life.

It is impossible to overemphasize the good that is being lost here. It is very immediate, tangible, and direct. It is the good of life itself, something that everyone believes is worth saving. Not only is saving lives an intrinsically good thing, but it is a morally commendable goal, against which few other goals stack up.

Life is precious. To allow it to be wasted, when simple changes in our medical-legal system could save it, is a tragedy of human making, not of divine fact. True, we didn't cause the diseases that destroyed the organs, but we continue to allow the system to operate that prevents lives from being saved. Even if we changed the system to allow only rewarded cadaveric donation, many lives would be saved. (Perhaps this is the only change we need to make for a few years, while we acquire data on how the change works and study unanticipated consequences.) . . .

Alternatives haven't worked

Lack of transplantable organs motivates surgeons to find ways around current limitations imposed by ethics and will continue to do so until there are enough organs. Like a flooding river, this urgent need keeps trying to find ways over, under, or around the various ethical dams that appear in its path. Consider the following three alternatives to offering financial incentives, all of which raise ethical problems, some more serious than those raised by the financial incentives we are considering.

First, proposals constantly surface to broaden the scope of eligible cadaveric donors. Most have failed, but surgeons keep trying to expand definitions of *dead person, nonperson,* and *never a person* to include young patients in persistent vegetative states, non-heart-beating donors (the controversial protocol originated at the University of Pittsburgh Medical Center, the transplant capital of the world), and anencephalic babies. Such changes in definition, generally practiced out of the light of public scrutiny and certainly without real public understanding, only increase public distrust of the transplant system.

Second, dying people who need transplantable organs are constantly promised that breakthroughs are coming in artificial hearts, xenografts, and tissue engineering. A little perspective helps evaluate those claims. For example, surgeon Christiaan Barnard predicted in 1968 that pig hearts would be routinely transplanted into humans within twenty years. Thirty-two years later, we are not much closer to performing such transplants, much less performing them "routinely." The artificial heart was a disaster, in some cases not even fitting into the empty cavity of the patient awaiting it. Almost fifteen years later, no breakthroughs have occurred to solve the essential medical problems that plagued such devices. And where tissue engineering has done a good job of producing skin and ears, producing a functional heart or liver is another matter.

Third, proposals abound to get around the problem of families of brain-dead patients refusing to give voluntary, informed consent for donation. These proposals include required request (the law in most states, applying to families of potential cadaveric donors) and mandated choice (required request of individuals before they become potential donors, e.g., when they renew driver's licenses). When tried, such proposals have not increased the frequency of organ donation.

At worst, some proposals to change the system are unethical. Consider *presumed consent,* tried in Europe, where laws presume citizens consent to be organ donors, unless they state otherwise. Why has such a system failed and been considered immoral? [According to Lloyd Cohen, author of *Increasing the Supply of Transplant Organs:*]

> the European model of "presumed consent". . . is fundamentally dishonest. Under this regime the decedent or his next of kin have the legal right and theoretical power to opt out of donation but no clear mechanism with which to do so. Absent a national recording scheme, the decedent himself will almost never have an occasion to make his wishes known to the authorities. And, even his next of kin may be unaware of their right to choose on his behalf, or when that choice arises, or how to make their wishes known.

Systems of presumed consent have failed to increase organ donation in Europe, and justifiably so. Most people believe that they have a property right in their bodies and that consent is necessary for the disposal of it. The law in some European countries allows physicians to simply commandeer organs without asking for consent of families, but most such physicians refuse to do so. . . .

Hypocritical and inconsistent

American medicine makes very few transplants available free to those without medical coverage, so it is hypocritical to maintain that our present system is not influenced by money. Isn't it also hypocritical that the only people *not* paid in the whole system of organ transplantation are the families of donors? Everyone else gets paid, and paid very well indeed. As the Bellagio Report on paid organ transplantation observed in 1997, "After-all, transplantation is hardly a commercial-free transaction. Hospitals, surgeons, organ retrieval teams and procurement organizations regularly sell their services. Why should the source of the organ be the only one not financially rewarded?"

As I said before, blood, eggs, semen, tissue, spines, and entire cadavers are already being sold. Why not then allow payment for kidneys from cadavers? As the Bellagio Report concluded in 1997:

> the sale of body parts is already so widespread that it is not self-evident why solid organs should be excluded. In many countries, blood, sperm, and ova may be sold. So too, an international trade exists in cadaveric body parts for medical education and research, and pharmaceutical companies purchase large quantities of tissue for commercial purposes. Other companies openly purchase and sell tissue such as dura mater and fascia lata.

Furthermore, people get a tax deduction for donating money for research to find a cure for AIDS or cancer. Isn't this a public policy that "rewards" giving a gift? A gift aimed at maximizing life?

One objection holds that it is permissible to allow payment for renewable bodily tissue but not for nonrenewable tissue. The Bellagio Report skewers this objection nicely:

> The counter-argument that unlike solid organs, blood and sperm are self-renewing body parts is not telling, for if the risk to health in selling one kidney is truly minimal (which it is, at least in developed countries), then much of the relevance of the distinction disappears. By the same token, on what grounds may blood or bone be traded on the open market but not cadaveric kidneys?

The right kind of motive

. . . Paying money to families to increase organ donation is considered immoral because it appeals to the wrong kind of motives in the people who consent. What is the right kind of motive? The answer, of course, is altruism. The official view in medicine, what I call *presumed altruism,* asserts that humans are altruistic and should give to one another unselfishly, especially when life itself is at stake. Clergy say that this is God's plan for helping mankind. Some philosophers and economists say that public policy must both assume some bit of altruism in humans and encourage it to flourish.

Presumed altruism is behind the position that the main reason why people don't donate is because of ignorance and, therefore, what we need is more education. In other words, people would donate if only they were educated enough about the need and lack of risks to themselves.

This position does not seem to be true. Over the past three decades, millions upon millions of dollars and thousands of persuasive pieces in the print and visual media have educated North Americans about the great need for organ donors, and indeed, large percentages of people in theory say they would donate. But when asked in actual cases, only a small percentage do.

What sane system allows thousands of good organs to go to the worms each year, when there are untried ways to increase organ donation?

So it seems that the present system is not working to meet demand. Put somewhat dramatically, no amount of pleading, of agonized chest-beating, of doleful pictures of dying children, seems likely to increase significantly the number of donated organs. Put more dramatically, we could ask what sane system allows thousands of good organs to go to the worms each year, when there are untried ways to increase organ donation? . . .

Morally wrong in itself

Offering financial incentives is most often said to be wrong because it makes commodities of humans, their bodies, or parts of the human body. This claim is made over and over again in the literature by surgeons and others. But such surgeons generally do not articulate why it was wrong to allow selling kidneys, they merely repeatedly say that it is "obviously" wrong.

Offering financial incentives for cadaveric donation is ethically justified and practical.

Consider the following summation of arguments against commercialization in one medical journal specializing in transplantation:

> [To permit payment for kidneys would be wrong because it would be] the commodification of the body; treating the body as an "it" rather than as a "self"; diminution of altruism in society at large; the coarsening of society's view of other persons; and so on. All these become a greater burden on society if human life is cheapened by putting a price on living human organs.

This typical argument is more assertion than reason. Consider another, similar summation:

> To market organs for transplantation, or any other purpose, would be to market pieces of the self, pieces of the person, to put a price on human life and health best thought of as priceless. [Moreover] . . . neither transplantation itself, nor efficiency in the supply of organs, should be viewed as goods worth any price. There is a widely shared perception, reflected in our laws and other public policies, that some things should not be allowed in the marketplace.

Most of the above-mentioned statements assert that it is wrong to think of a part of the body as something that could be sold and that it would be better if people were altruistic. Of course, such arguments always leave out the people who are dying for lack of a transplant. Moreover, the last quotation appeals to a "perception" of the wrongness of commercialization, yet one 1992 poll found that most Americans favor some sort of financial incentive to increase organ donation, especially from cadavers.

A variation of this argument holds that the human body is sacred and should not be "desecrated," that is, the human body is "the Temple of the Lord." Such a view implies that bodies should be left intact at death and not "violated" by surgeons. This view has a long history originating at the beginnings of anatomy in opposing vivisection. . . .

It is true that Christians believe in resurrection of the body, but surely they don't believe that the body resurrected is the body actually buried. Few Christians believe that their resurrected body will be the one with the severed spinal cord or the emaciated shell of their one hundred five-year-old body. Instead, they believe that God restores the body in Heaven to its youthful prime. Given that God is omnipotent, he surely can also restore any organs then that were removed to benefit others on earth. . . .

Time to give limited compensation a try

After all these considerations, I believe that a mixed commercial/altruistic system would be best for Americans. I also believe that offering financial incentives for cadaveric donation is ethically justified and practical. Instituting such a system would likely save thousands of American lives each year and cause little harm to living people.

At the very least, the government could offer one thousand dollars as a voucher, payable only to funeral homes for burial expenses. Such "in-kind" reimbursement systems may defuse the objection that "life" is being bought and sold or that it has a price tag.

Why not try this plan? Let's do empirical, not a priori, ethics and see if the experiment works. As mentioned, Pennsylvania plans to offer at least three hundred dollars for funeral expenses for cadaveric donations. Armchair critics, such as columnist Ellen Goodman, immediately cried that such payments were "cheapening life." It's better, I guess, that hundreds of people die than to "cheapen life."

In 1997, the Bellagio Report studied this same issue. Like me, its commissioners were perplexed that the universal condemnations by transplant surgeons "failed to provide a rationale for their position." Although the reasons for their condemnation "appeared self-evident" to the surgeons, it did not seem so to the commissioners.

These commissioners were not convinced that rewarded giving would be the end of the world: "[We] found no unarguable ethical principle that would justify a ban on the sale of organs under all circumstances." They concluded that a government-financed and government-regulated system of rewarded giving could work. As for the slippery slope, "a firm line can be maintained, between cadaveric and live donation, reducing the likelihood of moving down a slippery slope."

Here is my final idea: let's try a controlled experiment on a limited scale, say, in two states that are similar and with similar records of previous organ donation. In one state, we try rewarded cadaveric donation, funded by fees from automobile licenses and using skilled nurses and counselors to ask families to participate. In the other state, we do nothing new, and the state can serve as a true control. Why not try this test? What have we got to lose?

6

Compensating People for Organ Donation Is Unethical

Stephen G. Post

Stephen G. Post is a professor at the Center for Biomedical Ethics at Case Western Reserve University and the author of Inquiries in Bioethics.

The buying and selling of human organs violates human dignity. A system in which the poor are forced to earn money by selling their body parts to the rich is unethical. For example, there is already a black market for organs in India wherein the poor sell their spare kidneys to the wealthy. The libertarian idea that the human body is property that can be sold off is objectionable and contrary to most religious teachings. Finally, commerce in human organs would undercut the spirit of philanthropy that currently drives organ donation, and thus may actually exacerbate the organ shortage.

Should we allow competent adults to sell their organs and tissues? The libertarian view, with its doctrine that freedom is the highest value, constrained only by the prohibition against harm to others (the "harm principle") but not to self, would allow the sale of body parts. Even on this view, proponents stop short of condoning the sale of vital organs, for this would result in death, although the logic of libertarianism would seem to allow even this. Libertarians would not be justifying the potential sale of spare body parts if there were no demand. As biomedical science advances in areas such as reproductive technology, fetal tissue transplant and organ transplantation, market incentives appear to be one way in which supply might meet escalating demands.

There has been resistance to the commercialization of body parts. For example, the National Institutes of Health now funds research in fetal transplants for Parkinson's disease patients. The NIH is clear, however, that no pregnant woman can sell her fetus. NIH ethics guidelines assume that if financial incentives were allowed, poor women surely would be-

From "Organ Volunteers Serve Body Politic," by Stephen G. Post, *Insight on the News,* January 9, 1995. Copyright © 1995 by News World Communications, Inc. Reprinted with permission.

come pregnant in order to make money through aborting the fetus, optimally at the beginning of the second trimester when the fetus has developed sufficiently but still contains undifferentiated brain cells, and selling the fetus to physicians or to patients with neurodegenerative diseases.

The utility of fetal tissue transplant still is debated, particularly in light of other possible medical therapies under development. But imagine what could happen if fetal tissue transplants were to work effectively as a cure or partial cure for the diseases of Alzheimer's and diabetes. The demand quickly would reach into the tens of millions. Four million people in the United States have Alzheimer's disease, and the number will triple as the baby boomers become elderly. For the Parkinson's operation, at least three to four fetuses are needed per transplant (a dime-size hole is drilled into the top of the skull, and fetal brain cells are implanted on the outer brain surface). The libertarian proclaims "long live freedom," and in the meantime, the problems of poverty and of children having children are finally solved—a welfare conservative's dream. Caregivers for people with various dementing diseases might be liberated from a sea of diapers and nursing home payments.

A form of oppression

The critics of commercialization of the fetus quickly point to the injustice of it all: The poor become pregnant to earn money that ultimately comes from the wealthier classes. Surely a wealthy woman who is financially comfortable will not need to sell fetuses. A poor woman might be able to sell four fetuses a year, perhaps at several thousand dollars each. Perhaps the moral ambiguity of abortion will entirely disappear in a culture that establishes a new profession in fetal sales. While this is all rather futuristic, it should be remembered that in India, where a huge black market in nonvital body parts provides kidneys for the wealthy, it is the poor who sell. Is this truly freedom, as the libertarian proclaims? Or is it a forced choice made in destitution and contrary to the seller's true human nature? I see such a market as the most demeaning form of human oppression, as unworthy of any valid human freedom, and as reducing the unborn child to mere grist in the medical mill.

In addition to the risk of creating a class of oppressed sellers . . . there is a second specter associated with the market approach: low-quality parts.

The NIH rightly forbids the sale of fetuses, as well as the designation of particular fetal-tissue recipients such as a father or some other loved one, for fear of emotional pressure on the donor. Of course, even on the current basis of voluntary donation, many are disturbed by the very idea of encouraging the "harvesting" of fetuses as an act of beneficence, akin to donating blood. Will signs on buses read, "Be a giver of life. Donate your fetus today"?

Writing in 1971, Richard Titmuss lamented the commercialization of the blood supply in the United States. He wrote that "proportionately more blood is being supplied by the poor, the unskilled, the unemployed, Negroes and other low-income groups." He warned of a new class of exploited "high blood yielders" and of redistribution of blood from poor to rich. Fortunately, by 1982 only 3 to 4 percent of blood came from paid donors. Moreover, various social scientific studies indicated that the American people favored a voluntary system and were disturbed by the buying and selling of blood. Personal solicitation, coupled with more convenient donation opportunities, had proved to be highly effective.

In addition to the risk of creating a class of oppressed sellers (who might provide organs, bone marrow, blood and ova, in addition to fetuses), there is a second specter associated with the market approach: low-quality parts. Titmuss warned against the increasing danger to the American blood supply due to contagion. The sale of blood is forbidden by the American Red Cross because sales two decades ago included samples of blood from people infected with pathogens. Drug addicts, for example, routinely sold blood, thereby passing on diseases such as hepatitis. Because those who sell are inevitably the most needy and marginalized, the likelihood of contagion is great. The blood supply is now much purer because it relies entirely on volunteerism. Sperm is sold and must be carefully tested for contagion. Still, a small number of women have become HIV infected as a result of receiving tainted sperm. Spare parts, tissues and body fluids gathered for a fee are, on the whole, of poor quality.

Oppression of the poor and poor quality are concerns that fall under the moral rubric of "do no harm." There is another concern that involves not the avoidance of harm but the doing of good. When the call goes out to a community for bone marrow, blood or some other lifesaving bodily substance, the spirit of beneficence is tapped. Often, we discover within ourselves a moral idealism that serves the neighbor in the form of disinterested love. In an age of considerable greed and solipsism, the expression of connectedness with unknown others is a welcome sight. Volunteerism allows the community to express moral idealism when moral minimalism is the order of the day. The marketing of body parts undercuts and even eradicates one of the important implementations of the philanthropic conscience.

In 1994 this point was driven home to millions of Italians—their country has one of the world's lowest donation rates—by the selfless example of two American tourists. During a foiled robbery attempt, Italian bandits had killed the 7-year-old son of Reginald and Maggie Green of Bodega Bay, California. The decision by the couple to donate their son's organs stunned the nation as a gesture of extraordinary generosity and triggered an outpouring of organ donations.

The body is not property

Finally, there is the issue of human dignity and the body as property. In most religious traditions the body has not been perceived as a possession over which one has property rights. Instead, it has been interpreted as that over which we have stewardship. In general terms, human beings are responsible for their bodies as stewards or caretakers, but they do not own their bodies, which are ultimately the property of the creator. Hence, the classical argument against suicide in Western culture was always, "God giveth life, and God taketh away." The ultimate authority over the body and over bodily life is God, and that ought not to be usurped. In the most general terms, then, a sacred dimension to the body places limits on our human authority to "own" it. For this reason, Jewish, Roman Catholic and Protestant ethics emphasized the integrity of the body, the sin of self-mutilation and respectful treatment of the body even after death. Hence, when the first cornea transplants emerged, theologians seriously debated whether cornea procurement violates "integrity."

A sacred dimension to the body places limits on our human authority to "own" it.

Despite the success of transplantation during the last three decades, there are too few who donate body parts. This is largely because on some deep psychological level, human beings are reluctant to have themselves or their loved ones "picked apart." Medical anthropologists have long observed that Asian Pan-Confucianism, from China to Japan, forbids donating body parts because the body is bequeathed by one's ancestors, so that to mutilate it is to violate filial duties. Orthodox Judaism categorically condemns organ procurement from the living and the dead. On one hand, these traditions can be dismissed as archaic, to be set aside by rational, empirical, scientific progress. It appears, however, that they articulate a universal anxiety about taking such liberties with the body.

Enter here the libertarians. If spare parts are scarce, if no degree of appeal to beneficence seems to dramatically elevate the levels of procurement, then why not move past archaic anxieties by enlisting the almighty dollar? After all, people will do just about anything for money, even if they feel that they violate the body's moral demand for respect.

Commercialism undermines community

To some degree, we have succeeded in negotiating with tradition by creating a culture of giving and receiving body parts. True, there are organ shortages, but procurement is steady. To go from the reasonably successful moral idealism of generous giving and grateful receiving to selling and buying certainly undermines the spirit of community. Moreover, selling and buying may not even produce the desired results in increased supply. When blood procurement relied on selling, there was considerably less blood available than there is now. We have taken on highly symbolic meanings. Commercialization may repulse rather than entice.

True, commercialization has begun to emerge. Sperm, eggs and surrogate wombs are sold and bought. In India, the sale of a kidney ensures comfort for one's family. Before it is too late, I recommend a categorical ban on all sales of body parts in the U.S., and a renewed appeal to the philanthropic conscience that lies within us all, even if obscured by the ubiquity of the profit motive.

7

Research on Cloning Would Help Alleviate the Organ Shortage

Peter A. Brown

Peter A. Brown is an editorial page columnist for the Orlando Sentinel.

In November 2001, President George W. Bush called for a ban on research into human cloning. Such opposition to cloning research is based mostly on a belief that reproductive cloning is morally wrong. However, scientists are years away from being able to clone cells that will mature into a viable baby. Instead, cloning research is likely to first yield ways of cloning cells and growing them into specific organs, such as a heart or kidney, rather than living persons. Cloning research should not be banned because of far-fetched scenarios; instead it should be pursued because it could alleviate the organ shortage and save countless lives.

Everyone from President Bush to the pope is clamoring to ban the cloning of human embryos. That, itself, might be reason to consider whether the opposition is based on well-considered arguments or simple fear of the scientific unknown.

Some fear people will be manufactured in laboratories, as dramatized by the 1978 film "The Boys from Brazil," in which renegade scientists tried to clone Adolf Hitler.

Test-tube babies come to mind when people think human cloning, even though the more likely use would be to combat disease and produce designer organs that would reduce rejection and eliminate the current waiting list for transplants.

A divisive issue

But, let's put aside the science for a moment. The questions over cloning are as much political, economic and moral. The answers are complicated, because the issue forces us to make choices among deeply held beliefs.

From "Cloning Is Worth the Risk," by Peter A. Brown, *Knight-Ridder/Tribune News Service*, December 3, 2001. Copyright © 2001 by Knight-Ridder/Tribune News Service. Reprinted with permission.

Philosophically, the question is about how much government should restrict the private sector, and whether heartfelt views about morality should play a role in that decision. Yet, isn't the key issue whether government should protect us from scientific progress?

European Research Commissioner Philippe Busquin framed the issue with a candor not likely to be heard from U.S. officials committed to free-market capitalism and limited government unknown in the European Union. "Not everything scientifically possible, and technologically feasible, is necessarily desirable or admissible," he said.

[Cloning research] could produce designer hearts, livers and kidneys that would both alleviate the growing shortage of human organs for transplantation, [and] greatly reduce the chances of organ rejection.

He may be right, but those seeking to capitalize on public discomfort might want to consider this corollary: Government should not restrict every activity that might be politically unpopular if public money isn't used.

Otherwise, government essentially would be picking scientific winners and losers, a role it has declined in fostering economic innovation. The marketplace, not politicians, should pick those winners.

In some ways, the issue is a more complicated version of the abortion debate, asking whether a person's or politicians' moral values should guide public policy governing an issue on which honorable people differ.

The head of the Massachusetts company that cloned the embryos said he would not transplant them into a woman's womb to produce a baby. There are also serious questions whether this process could produce a viable baby, while the chance that cloned cells could successfully produce scarce organs appears to be greater.

The House of Representatives last summer [2000] passed a bill that would ban cloning, whether used for medical purposes and creating a new source of organs for transplantation, or to create human beings. But until the cloning announcement Sunday [November 27, 2001, in which President Bush urged Congress to pass the proposed ban on human cloning], the issue sat on the Senate back-burner.

Clearly, it is the prospect of mad scientists creating new human beings that makes people the most uncomfortable. However, one person's mad scientist is the next one's Nobel Prize nominee.

But lost in the frenzy to rein in cloning is the bigger question: Five, 10 or 20 years from now, will the world be better off with such research?

After all, if scientists could clone Hitler, as "The Boys from Brazil" depicted as a plot to resurrect the Nazi regime, then why not Albert Einstein, who could provide countless new scientific breakthroughs?

Moreover, worth considering is whether the current furor is any different than two decades ago when babies were first produced through in-vitro fertilization. Critics warned it would threaten the sanctity of human life, but these days it is an accepted medical procedure that allows once-childless couples to become parents.

It is in this context that few seemingly want to consider whether the potential abuses of human-cloning work are worrisome enough to outweigh the potential medical benefits.

Designer organs

In the long run, this work could produce designer hearts, livers and kidneys that would both alleviate the growing shortage of human organs for transplantation, but greatly reduce the chances of organ rejection.

The scientific genie is out of the bottle. No matter what government does, it can't stop the inevitable development of this technology. Nor should it. Regardless of what lawmakers do, work will continue underground and offshore.

There are legitimate reasons to be concerned about the abuses that cloning could create. Millions of Americans hold moral/religious beliefs that make cloning unacceptable to them.

That is their right. But it's another question whether they should impose their beliefs on those who do not share them. That is what they would be doing by having the law limit research they find morally repugnant.

Using Cloned Humans for Organ Transplants Would Be Unethical

Charles Krauthammer

Charles Krauthammer is a Pulitzer Prize–winning columnist for the
Washington Post.

Several scientists have posited that cloning technology could one
day be used to grow headless humans in the laboratory. These
creatures, they argue, would lack sentience and therefore be ideal
sources for organs. This idea of creating human mutants to serve
as organ donors is abhorrent and shows how cloning technology
might be abused. Human cloning should be banned, and the deliberate creation of headless humans should be made a crime.

The ultimate cloning horror: human organ farms
Last year [1997] Dolly the cloned sheep was received with wonder, tit-
ters and some vague apprehension. . . . The announcement by a Chicago
physicist that he is assembling a team to produce the first human clone
occasioned yet another wave of *Brave New World* [the title of the 1932
novel by Aldous Huxley in which all humans are cloned—not born—into
specific social classes] anxiety. But the scariest news of all—and largely
overlooked—comes from two obscure labs, at the University of Texas and
at the University of Bath. During the past four years, one group created
headless mice; the other, headless tadpoles.

For sheer Frankenstein wattage, the purposeful creation of these animal monsters has no equal. Take the mice. Researchers found the gene
that tells the embryo to produce the head. They deleted it. They did this
in a thousand mice embryos, four of which were born. I use the term
loosely. Having no way to breathe, the mice died instantly.

Why then create them? The Texas researchers want to learn how
genes determine embryo development. But you don't have to be a genius
to see the true utility of manufacturing headless creatures: for their organs—fully formed, perfectly useful, ripe for plundering.

From "Of Headless Mice . . . and Men: The Ultimate Cloning Horror: Human Organ Farms," by
Charles Krauthammer, *Time,* January 19, 1998. Copyright © 1998 by Time, Inc. Reprinted with
permission.

Why should you be panicked? Because humans are next. "It would almost certainly be possible to produce human bodies without a forebrain," Princeton biologist Lee Silver told the *London Sunday Times*. "These human bodies without any semblance of consciousness would not be considered persons, and thus it would be perfectly legal to keep them 'alive' as a future source of organs."

There is no grosser corruption of biotechnology than creating a human mutant and disemboweling it at our pleasure for spare parts.

"Alive." Never have a pair of quotation marks loomed so ominously. Take the mouse-frog technology, apply it to humans, combine it with cloning, and you become a god: with a single cell taken from, say, your finger, you produce a headless replica of yourself, a mutant twin, arguably lifeless, that becomes your own personal, precisely tissue-matched organ farm.

There are, of course, technical hurdles along the way. Suppressing the equivalent "head" gene in man. Incubating tiny infant organs to grow into larger ones that adults could use. And creating artificial wombs (as per Aldous Huxley), given that it might be difficult to recruit sane women to carry headless fetuses to their birth/death.

It won't be long, however, before these technical barriers are breached. The ethical barriers are already cracking. Lewis Wolpert, professor of biology at University College, London, finds producing headless humans "personally distasteful" but, given the shortage of organs, does not think distaste is sufficient reason not to go ahead with something that would save lives. And Professor Silver not only sees "nothing wrong, philosophically or rationally," with producing headless humans for organ harvesting; he wants to convince a skeptical public that it is perfectly O.K.

When prominent scientists are prepared to acquiesce in—or indeed encourage—the deliberate creation of deformed and dying quasi-human life, you know we are facing a bioethical abyss. Human beings are ends, not means. There is no grosser corruption of biotechnology than creating a human mutant and disemboweling it at our pleasure for spare parts.

The prospect of headless human clones should put the whole debate about "normal" cloning in a new light. Normal cloning is less a treatment for infertility than a treatment for vanity. It is a way to produce an exact genetic replica of yourself that will walk the earth years after you're gone.

But there is a problem with a clone. It is not really you. It is but a twin, a perfect John Doe Jr., but still a junior. With its own independent consciousness, it is, alas, just a facsimile of you.

The headless clone solves the facsimile problem. It is a gateway to the ultimate vanity: immortality. If you create a real clone, you cannot transfer your consciousness into it to truly live on. But if you create a headless clone of just your body, you have created a ready source of replacement parts to keep you—your consciousness—going indefinitely.

Which is why one form of cloning will inevitably lead to the other. Cloning is the technology of narcissism, and nothing satisfies narcissism like immortality. Headlessness will be cloning's crowning achievement.

The time to put a stop to this is now. Dolly moved President Bill Clinton to create a commission that recommended a temporary ban on human cloning. But with physicist Richard Seed threatening to clone humans, and with headless animals already here, we are past the time for toothless commissions and meaningless bans.

Clinton banned federal funding of human-cloning research, of which there is none anyway. He then proposed a five-year ban on cloning. This is not enough. Congress should ban human cloning now. Totally. And regarding one particular form, it should be draconian: the deliberate creation of headless humans must be made a crime, indeed a capital crime. If we flinch in the face of this high-tech barbarity, we'll deserve to live in the hell it heralds.

9

Patients Should Be Allowed to Permit the Removal of Their Organs Shortly After Death

James M. DuBois

James M. DuBois is a medical doctor and associate professor of health care ethics at St. Louis University.

Most organs for transplant come from donors who suffer a sudden death after a traumatic head injury. This allows physicians to quickly declare the patients' death and remove organs before they are damaged. However, most people die more slowly—by the time physicians declare the patients dead, their organs are not suitable for transplant. Proposals to give doctors more flexibility in determining time of death raise fears that doctors may rush to declare death in order to procure organs from donors. However, it may be possible to design a system in which patients on life support give their permission for doctors to remove their organs shortly after life support is removed and death occurs.

O rgan donation after death is considered a generous gift, a gift of life. In harmony with many religious traditions, the Catholic Church teaches that organ donation can be a concrete gesture of "solidarity and self-giving love" and "meritorious." Yet many people cannot donate organs because of the circumstances of their death. Aside from living donation (most typically of a single kidney), solid organ donation requires that the organs be procured after the donor has died but before the transplantable organs have themselves died.

Most organ donors are declared dead after a traumatic head injury. Such circumstances permit attending physicians to use neurological (or brain death) criteria to declare the donors dead, even while the donors' circulation and respiration are being maintained artificially. However,

From "Non-Heart-Beating Organ Donation: Designing an Ethically Acceptable Protocol," by James M. DuBois, *Health Progress*, January/February 2001. Copyright © 2001 by the Catholic Health Association of the United States. Reprinted with permission.

this pool of organ donors has always been inadequate to meet need. Moreover, most people do not die from traumatic injury and thus cannot donate organs after death even though they might have wanted to do so.

Non–heart-beating organ donation (NHBD) provides an alternative for some patients. In this article I will focus only on "controlled" NHBD, in which patients or their proxies decide to withdraw life support because life support is futile or excessively burdensome. NHBD protocols use circulatory-respiratory (CR) criteria to determine death. The unusual twist to NHBD protocols is that death must be declared within a few minutes after CR functions are lost; otherwise solid organs are severely damaged by warm ischemia (lack of oxygenation at body temperature). NHBD protocols give rise to many ethical questions. Nevertheless, the use of a well-designed NHBD protocol is ethically acceptable. With this article, I hope to help hospitals identify the major ethical issues so that they may design an acceptable protocol while providing an adequate ethical rationale to the public.

Protecting donor interests

Using a person merely as a means to an end is wrong. Put otherwise, acting against one person's dignity for the sake of another is wrong. In the context of organ donation, this principle requires that the organ donor always be shown respect. The benefit to the organ recipient, great as that may be, does not justify harming the donor—even in the last minutes of life. With these thoughts in mind, I will briefly touch on the most important donor safeguards that NHBD protocols should include.

How can one be sure that dead donors are really dead? The transplant community frequently speaks of the "dead donor rule." Laws and norms against homicide require that donors of vital organs not be killed in the process of procuring their organs. Some commentators claim that this is *all* the rule entails. In practice, the dead donor rule is usually understood to entail that vital organs not be procured until after death has been determined (even though, in some scenarios, organ procurement might not be the cause of death).

Most people do not die from traumatic injury and thus cannot donate organs after death even though they might have wanted to do so.

The U.S. Uniform Determination of Death Act of 1983 (UDDA) says death may be declared when a person sustains "either (1) irreversible cessation of circulatory and respiratory functions, or (2) irreversible cessation of all functions of the entire brain, including the brain stem." Although the presidential commission report on which the UDDA was based permits two different kinds of criteria to be used in determining death, it maintains that death is a unified phenomenon: the loss of integrative unity. Some commentators argue that NHBD patients are not dead because one must wait at least 9 or 10 minutes after cardiac arrest to establish that the donor's brain has incurred damage severe enough to meet brain death criteria. But this approach is mistaken. NHBD protocols use CR criteria, not neurological criteria, to determine death. This approach is consistent with defining death as a unified phenomenon: With the loss of CR functions, integrative unity is lost, the brain stops functioning, and consciousness is lost. Moreover, assuming that CR functions are *irreversibly* lost, all other functions (including brain functions) are irreversibly lost as well.

The dead donor rule is usually understood to entail that vital organs not be procured until after death has been determined.

Controversy also exists over competing interpretations of the UDDA requirement that functional losses be irreversible. NHBD protocols vary across the nation, but many state that death can be declared just two minutes after the patient's CR functions have ceased. We know, however, that aggressive cardiopulmonary resuscitation can often restore CR functions, even after two minutes of arrest. How can NHBD protocols then satisfy the legal requirements for irreversibility? Well-designed protocols do this by noting two facts:
- Available medical evidence suggests that no patient can revive without help (auto-resuscitate) two minutes or more following the cessation of CR functions.
- NHBD becomes an option only after a decision has been made to withdraw life support. Therefore, applying resuscitative measures would violate the patient's wishes as expressed in a valid do-not-resuscitate order.

The loss of CR function is both *naturally* and *morally* irreversible in such cases. If nature is allowed to take its course (and we are obliged to let it do so), function will not return. In waiting out a two-minute absence of pulse and breath, physicians are ensuring that the donor, being dead, will not be harmed by procurement.

Should heparin be administered before death is declared? NHBD protocols frequently instruct physicians to administer a large dose of the drug heparin after life support has begun to be withdrawn but before death is declared. Heparin is an anticoagulant used to ensure a proper "flush" of newly procured organs so that they may be preserved for transplantation. Some ethicists argue that heparin should not be administered routinely. Many patients who donate using NHBD protocols have head injuries. In such cases, an anticoagulant could cause massive brain hemorrhaging and death.

Is the premortem use of heparin unethical? Or can the principle of double effect be invoked? Certainly this scenario meets most of the requirements for the correct application of the double-effect principle. The physician's intention—thinning blood to ensure organ viability for transplant—is legitimate. The intention is not to hasten or cause the donor's death. Nor is the risk of death a means of achieving the good that is sought. Because, moreover, the patient has withdrawn life support and is in the process of dying, the good at stake is proportionate to any risk.

The objection some ethicists have to invoking the double-effect principle in such cases is this: Ordinarily the person who suffers the potential harm is also the beneficiary of the intended resulting good. These ethicists claim that since the organ recipient is the sole beneficiary of the use of heparin, the principle of double effect cannot be invoked. However, it is also possible to argue that, if the organ donor truly wanted to donate organs for the sake of another, enabling him or her to realize this wish is a good for the donor. If this rationale is accepted, then the uniform use of heparin before death may be justified.

Of course, the principle of double effect also requires that the action be necessary to bring about the good. Some transplant teams, having questioned the uniform use of heparin before death is determined, are exploring other options: administering heparin immediately after death is declared, for example, or using a cold perfusion technique as an alternative. The Institute of Medicine (IOM) wisely recommends making such decisions on a case-by-case basis. It also urges transplant teams to obtain informed consent for the use of any medication that does not directly benefit the donor.

Avoiding conflicts of interest

NHBD, like all forms of organ donation, presents potential conflicts of interest that must be avoided to protect the interests of donors and their families. NHBD protocols should address at least four possible conflicts of interest.

The decision to discontinue treatment must come first. The issue of donation should not be raised until the potential donor or his or her family has decided to discontinue treatment. In the early years of NHBD, some protocols prohibited medical personnel from raising the issue of donation; NHBD protocols were to be used only if the family raised the donation issue. Naturally great sensitivity must be shown to families when broaching the subject of organ donation, but NHBD presents no unique obstacles to making the request. One should simply wait until after a decision has been made to withdraw life support, thereby avoiding conflicts of interest.

Medical treatment and organ procurement must be kept separate. The physician who makes the determination of death cannot be a member of the transplant team.

The issue of donation should not be raised until the potential donor or his or her family has decided to discontinue treatment.

Donation costs must not fall on the donor family. The family should incur no expenses related to the donation process. NHBD protocols typically state that, should the potential donor not die within 30 to 60 minutes after withdrawing life support, he or she will be returned to the intensive care unit and the family will resume responsibility for expenses incurred thereafter.

Donors must receive standard-of-care treatment. In the well-publicized University of Pittsburgh NHBD protocol, donors were not given morphine or comfort care unless they visibly showed signs of distress. This practice was an effort to avoid the impression that morphine was used to hasten death. Ironically, it may have sacrificed patient interests in an effort to avoid giving the impression of doing so; as a result, the University of Pittsburgh team has since changed the practice. If patients at a given hospital routinely receive comfort care during the process of withdrawing life support, then this same standard should be adopted in the NHBD protocol.

Obligations to organ recipients

Although ethical discussions about organ transplantation tend to focus on organ donors, we have ethical obligations to organ recipients as well. Above all, we need to guarantee these patients that we will do everything we reasonably can to make their transplant a success. To do that, we must ensure that the transplantable organ is sufficiently healthy.

We have a duty not to damage the reputation of organ donation by offending members of the public.

The 1997 IOM report cites evidence that success rates with organs procured from NHBD donors and brain-dead donors are comparable. However, they are comparable because certain safeguards are standard. For example, if potential NHBD donors do not die within 30 to 60 minutes after the removal of life support, they are declared ineligible as donors. This is done largely because, although such patients' circulation may not have ceased entirely, their organs are in most cases poorly perfused during withdrawal of life support and have begun to die. Similarly, future data may show that NHBD requires the use of heparin or cannulation (the insertion of tubes for cold perfusion) before death.

Obligations to donor families

Cadaveric organ donation occurs at times that are already stressful and emotionally painful for donors' families, and NHBD presents some unique challenges for them.

Family members frequently want to be with their dying loved one. They want to be present when death is declared. Yet NHBD requires that organ procurement begin minutes after death is declared. In such cases, life support is therefore often withdrawn in the operating room (OR), after the body has been prepped for surgery. Most people would not choose this environment for a loved one to die in. Medical personnel need to be sensitive to this fact.

NHBD protocols frequently permit families to remain in the OR until the moment the donor dies. Family members are informed well in advance why they need to leave the OR quickly after the determination of death. There is no perfect way to deal with this challenge. But some hospitals are creative: When their floor layouts permit it, they allow the family to wait with the patient in a room near the OR until the declaration of death is made, thereby accommodating family wishes.

As noted, donor families should be protected from incurring financial expenses of the organ donation process. Their exemption from such responsibility should be explicitly stated in the consent process and in the NHBD protocol.

Developing protocols

NHBD protocols are typically crafted by and for local communities. Most NHBD protocol committees include lay persons, religious leaders or clergy, ethicists, and sometimes members of the local media. This approach gives protocol committees an opportunity to gain community input, approval, and oversight.

However, the approach has disadvantages. Lay people are, for example, not experts on many of the medical and ethical issues involved in NHBD. A committee that recruits members who lack authority to make decisions may create a false appearance of oversight and consensus; but a committee that gives each of its members—even the inexpert—equal authority may be acting irresponsibly. Moreover, the current habit of basing protocols on local practice guarantees that the protocols will vary in significant respects: Some allow the use of heparin, for example, whereas others do not; some require a wait of five minutes or more after CR function loss, whereas others require only that CR functions cease. Because such disparities have the potential to create scandal, they certainly do not reflect a strong commitment to ethical or medical best practice.

The IOM, in both its 1997 and 2000 reports, urges transplant committees to follow certain standard guidelines. Although not all legally binding, these guidelines provide committees with certain advantages:

- They reflect the consensus of panels of experts involved in NHBD.
- Should NHBD cause ethical concern in a particular community, the fact that local committees are following IOM-sanctioned guidelines may help allay that concern.

Fear and public opinion

We have a duty not to damage the reputation of organ donation by offending members of the public. In drafting protocols, NHBD committees should ask themselves not only, "Is this ethical and humane?" but also "Will it be *perceived* as ethical and humane?" Committees generally understand that even if administering heparin (for example) is not intrinsically wrong, it will become wrong if the scandal it creates hurts organ donation rates. This insight is basically sound.

However, like many other ethical norms, those concerning NHBD must be balanced. Protocol committees need to build an ethical rationale into certain aspects of their protocol. NHBD protocols should be public documents, and they should provide accounts of prescribed actions. But once we have constructed a solid ethical rationale, we should refuse to allow fear to drive our actions and interfere with medical best practice.

10
Vital Organs Must Never Be Removed from Patients Before Death

John A. Robertson

John A. Robertson is a professor at the University of Texas law school, where he teaches criminal law and bioethics. He is the author of Children of Choice: Freedom and the New Reproductive Technologies.

One of the most important ethical rules surrounding organ transplants is the "dead donor rule," which states that donors may not be killed in order to obtain their organs. Some exceptions to this rule have been proposed. First, some hospitals have proposed harvesting organs from anencephalic infants (who are born without an upper brain) in order to save other infants. Second, some states have introduced bills that would allow death row prisoners to have their vital organs removed as a form of execution. These proposed exceptions to the dead donor rule are unlikely to be accepted by the public because of the dead donor rule's importance in ensuring that organ donation is a lifesaving, rather than a death-causing, act.

A lthough living persons donate kidneys, cadaveric donors are the main source of solid organs for transplantation. Yet cadaveric donations have never been sufficient to meet the needs of persons with end-stage organ disease. One factor among many that limits the availability of cadaveric organs is the dead donor rule—the ethical and legal rule that requires that donors not be killed in order to obtain their organs.

Laws and norms against homicide forbid killings done for any purpose, including killings done to obtain organs to save the life of others. These laws and norms apply even if the person is unconscious, extremely debilitated, or very near death. The effect is to create the dead donor rule—the rule that states that organ retrieval itself cannot cause death. Removal of organs necessary for life prior to demise would violate the dead donor rule regardless of the condition or consent of the donor be-

Excerpted from "The Dead Donor Rule," by John A. Robertson, *Hastings Center Report,* November 1999. Copyright © 1999 by the Hastings Center. Reprinted with permission.

cause removal of those organs would kill the donor. Removal of nonvital organs prior to death would not violate the rule, though it would implicate other laws and ethical norms.

Laws and norms against killing are most clearly applicable when the person killed has not consented to the killing. But they also apply when a person requests death, whether to avoid suffering or to provide organs for transplant. The dead donor rule would thus prevent a person from committing suicide in order to provide organs to his family or others. In the short run the rule is deontologic rather than utilitarian, for it prevents the killing of one person for organs that would save the three or more lives that can be saved by a single cadaveric donor.

The dead donor rule . . . states that organ retrieval itself cannot cause death.

The dead donor rule is a center piece of the social order's commitment to respect for persons and human life. It is also the ethical linchpin of a voluntary system of organ donation, and helps maintain public trust in the organ procurement system. Although it is possible that some changes in the dead donor rule could be adopted without a major reduction in protection of persons and public trust, changes in the rule should be measured by their effect on both those functions.

Several recent proposals to increase the supply of cadaveric organs would create exceptions to the dead donor rule to allow donation when the donor lacks an upper brain and will imminently die (anencephalic infants) or will be executed (death row prisoners). These proposals do not challenge the rule's core function of protecting persons against unwanted demise. They do not, for example, propose a "survival lottery" in which persons are picked by chance to be killed to provide organs to several others. Nor would they permit competent persons to choose suicide by organ retrieval in order to save others. Instead, they would modify the rule at the margins of human life.

Proposals to permit donation from anencephalic infants or condemned prisoners aim to maintain respect for the core values underlying the dead donor rule while concluding that the benefits of relaxing the rule in these marginal cases outweigh the loss in respect for life and trust in the transplant system that might result. In contrast, proposals to retrieve organs from non-heart-beating donors claim to respect the dead donor rule as such by permitting organ retrieval only after the donor has been pronounced dead on cardiopulmonary grounds. Ethical controversy arises there, however, because uncertainties in determining cardiopulmonary death create a risk that the donor will not be dead when organ retrieval occurs, but will die as a result of the retrieval itself.

A closely related question concerns whether it is ethically acceptable for physicians to implement proposals that violate the dead donor rule in these marginal cases. From the time of Hippocrates, codes of medical ethics have condemned killing by physicians. This tradition continues strongly today in medical, ethical, and legal opposition to active euthanasia, physician-assisted suicide, and the participation of physicians in capital punishment and torture. If the dead donor rule is relaxed to facilitate organ procurement in these marginal cases, it will require a concomitant relaxation in prohibitions against physicians killing. Many persons would count such a change as an additional reason for opposing exceptions to the dead donor rule.

Respect prior to death for incompetent persons and those near death

The dead donor rule limits only organ retrieval that causes death. It says nothing about situations in which organ retrieval itself would not cause death. Removing nonessential organs or tissue from incompetent persons on the basis of substituted consent—for example, retrieving kidneys from retarded individuals or from those in persistent vegetative states—would not violate the dead donor rule because organ or tissue retrieval in those cases would not cause death. Retrieval of nonessential organs would, however, implicate concerns about showing proper respect for the dignity and well-being of incompetent persons, for example, not treating them as mere means to the ends of others. Although it would not violate the dead donor rule, retrieval in such cases still could not occur unless applicable ethical and legal requirements for consent by the donor or family had been met.

Some persons have mistakenly viewed the dead donor rule as also prohibiting retrieval of nonessential organs from comatose or incompetent persons prior to their death because ordinarily such organs are removed only after death has occurred. The fact that organ and tissue retrieval usually occurs after death, however, does not mean that retrieval cannot occur before death if ethical and legal norms for what may be done to persons prior to their death are observed.

The dead donor rule is a center piece of the social order's commitment to respect for persons and human life.

An example that nicely illustrates the distinction between the dead donor rule and rules for respecting incompetent persons would arise in a situation in which a family member, say the father, would like to donate a kidney to his daughter who suffers from end-stage kidney disease and who is not tolerating dialysis well. Medical examination shows that he has a serious heart condition that rules him out as a live donor. Soon after, he suffers a massive cardiac arrest that leaves him in a permanent coma in which he can be maintained indefinitely. At this point, removal of a kidney from him for transplantation to his daughter would not violate the dead donor rule because it would not cause his death. Whether it is ethically and legally acceptable, however, would depend on whether removal is consistent with laws and norms for respecting the interests of incompetent persons. In this case, based on his prior expressed wishes to donate to his daughter and the absence of harm to him from the donation, a plausible claim can be made that removal of the kidney is ethically and legally acceptable. If this option were not acceptable to the family, they could request that he be treated as a non-heart-beating donor, that is, have life support stopped, and then retrieve his kidney after he has been pronounced dead.

A key factor in observing the dead donor rule is the determination of death. The United States and most European countries now accept that death can be determined by tests that show irreversible cessation of circulatory and respiratory function or irreversible cessation of all functions of the entire brain. The latter tests—tests for whole-brain death—are necessary when the irreversible cessation of cardiopulmonary functions in a mechanically assisted patient cannot be independently established. . . .

Anencephalic infants

One proposal to change the dead donor rule would allow the retrieval of vital organs from anencephalic infants before they have suffered whole-brain death. Because few children die in circumstances where brain death is pronounced, organs for pediatric transplant, where organ size is a crucial factor, are in very short supply. Faced with the shortage of pediatric hearts, one center tried unsuccessfully to transplant a heart from a baboon to an infant with hypoplastic heart disease. Because of medical and ethical opposition to further use of xenografts, the center then proposed with parental consent to use organs from anencephalic newborns who had expired after treatment was withdrawn. When it was found that viable organs could not be obtained from anencephalic infants after death, consideration turned to removing organs before brain stem activity had ceased.

Such an alternative, however, is blocked by the dead donor rule. Although anencephalics lack an upper brain, they do have brain stem function, and thus are legally alive under existing criteria and tests for whole-brain death. Removing hearts and livers from anencephalic infants prior to total brain death would thus violate the dead donor rule and could be punishable as homicide. If anencephalics were to be a viable source of organs for pediatric transplant, an exception to the dead donor rule would have to be enacted into law and incorporated into ethical norms. . . .

Removing hearts and livers from anencephalic infants prior to total brain death would . . . violate the dead donor rule.

Strong arguments . . . exist against recognizing an exception. A primary one is the need to keep a bright line against killing individuals who are alive. Opponents also cite the difficulties in diagnosing anencephaly and the corresponding risk of mistaken diagnoses, the small number of children who would benefit, and the risk that this exception would make it much more likely that additional exceptions to the dead donor rule would be enacted for those in persistent vegetative states or with severe, irreversible mental illnesses. An exception might also reinforce public fears that the interests of organ donors would be sacrificed to obtain organs, and violate symbolic concerns for showing respect for human life by not killing. Finally, physicians would, in the very act of retrieving vital organs, be killing the anencephalic patient.

The arguments against recognizing an exception to the dead donor rule for anencephalic infants have carried the day. For example, the favorable 1992 opinion of the Council on Ethical and Judicial Affairs of the American Medical Association was withdrawn in the face of wide opposition and never reissued. . . .

Bills to permit organ retrievals from executions have been introduced in a few state legislatures.

An additional factor conserving the dead donor rule in the case of anencephalic infants is the necessity for the government openly to authorize a change in the definition of death or in the law of homicide to allow killing by organ retrieval of anencephalic infants. Even if legal immunity from prosecution were provided, medical opposition to physicians removing organs that cause an anencephalic child's death might still continue. Indeed, transplant physicians might refuse to retrieve or use organs from anencephalics to prevent erosion of public trust in the organ donation and transplant system. . . .

Organ retrieval as a form of execution

With over 3,200 persons now awaiting execution in the United States and some forty to seventy-five prisoners executed each year, proposals to retrieve organs for transplant from capital punishment have surfaced in recent years. The idea gained slight momentum in the early 1990s when a condemned prisoner in Georgia offered to donate organs as part of his execution and sued unsuccessfully for the opportunity. Bills to permit organ retrievals from executions have been introduced in a few state legislatures.

In considering proposals to use the organs of condemned prisoners, we must distinguish procuring organs from executed prisoners after their death or during their lives from procuring organs from them as a form of execution. There is no ethical or legal objection to removing organs or tissue from executed bodies after death, if consent of the deceased or next of kin has been obtained. Although most methods of execution would render organs unacceptable for transplant, the unclaimed bodies of executed inmates are routinely given to medical schools for anatomical study. Nor is there any ethical bar to a condemned prisoner serving as a living donor of a kidney or tissue, as long as the prisoner freely consents. Indeed, Texas and other capital punishment states permit live donations from condemned prisoners.

The question of execution by organ retrieval is quite different. To avoid the damaging effects on organs from execution by lethal injection, electrocution, hanging, gas, or firing squad, organ retrieval itself would become the method of execution. The condemned prisoner would request this method five to seven days before the execution date. At the time selected for execution, the prisoner would be taken from death row to the prison hospital and strapped on a gurney as in preparation for execution by lethal injection. Witnesses to the execution, including the victim's family, could view the insertion of intravenous lines and administration of anesthetic outside of the operating room. When the prisoner became unconscious, he would be moved to an operating room where the transplant team would then remove all his organs. When organ removal was completed, ventilatory or other mechanical assistance would be terminated, as occurs in retrieval from brain-dead, heart-beating cadavers. Death would be pronounced as having occurred either at the time that the heart and lungs were removed, or when mechanical assistance was terminated. The retrieved organs would then be distributed to consenting recipients in accordance with existing rules for distributing organs.

Such a procedure would clearly violate the dead donor rule. Retrieval of vital organs itself would be the cause of death because once heart, lungs, and liver are removed one would soon have to turn off the heart-lung bypass machines that are sustaining function during removal of vital organs. Physicians retrieving organs would thus also be executing the prisoner. For such a procedure to be acceptable, an exception to the dead donor rule in the case of executions would have to be recognized.

The main argument for an exception in this case is that the prisoner will in any case be executed. An exception to the rule to permit a mode of execution that protects organs would not harm the prisoner or deprive him of continued life, and thus would not infringe or deny the core values underlying the dead donor rule. The state in any case will be executing the prisoner, and the exception would permit the state to kill another in a way that salvages his organs. In addition, an exception for execution by organ retrieval has the salutary effect of respecting and preserving the lives of recipients at the very moment that the condemned person's life is taken as punishment for his having previously taken the life of others. . . .

The opponents of execution by organ retrieval have prevailed, and are likely to prevail for some time to come. The great aversion to an exception to the dead donor rule in the case of lawful executions is not adequately explained by the values underlying the dead donor rule. If state employees may legally kill a condemned criminal by drug, gas, or more violent means, it should not matter that execution occurs by removal of vital organs. This would not constitute an unconstitutional "cruel or unusual" punishment because there is nothing crueler about this method of execution, chosen by the prisoner, than other methods.

The opponents of execution by organ retrieval have prevailed, and are likely to prevail for some time to come.

A stronger ground for opposition is the role that transplant physicians and nurses would necessarily play in a system of execution by organ retrieval. Execution by organ retrieval could not be carried out by non-physician executioners as now occurs with execution by lethal injection and other methods. Even if some transplant doctors and nurses who accept the moral validity of capital punishment might be willing to participate in organ retrieval executions, their participation would violate medical ethical pronouncements against the participation of physicians in executions. The execution would also have to occur in the operating room of a hospital. If the prison hospital lacked adequate facilities, a hospital willing to allow organ retrieval executions on its premises would have to be found—and it is likely that few transplant teams or hospitals would be willing to participate.

The use of NHBDs involves: no violation of the dead donor rule and requires no public alteration or exception to it.

Opposition to such an exception also arises from the need to keep the death penalty separate from other social institutions. The death penalty is highly problematic morally, legally, and socially in those states that allow it; it would become even more so if it also served as a method of organ procurement. Interjecting transplantation into the controversy over capital punishment could also taint public perceptions of the beneficence of transplantation. Members of the public might come to view organ procurement teams as "killers" who harvest organs before or after death. Such a perception could reduce the willingness of families to donate, and thus impair the prospects of persons awaiting transplants. The purpose and effect of capital punishment is to end the life of a person who has himself taken life. Trying at the same time to preserve other lives through execution by organ retrieval only confuses the situation. It is best for organ transplantation and capital punishment to go their separate ways.

Non-heart-beating donors

Another proposal to increase the supply of cadaveric organs for transplant focusing attention on the dead donor rule is the use of non-heart-beating cadavers as organ donors. The first cadaveric organ donors were persons declared dead on cardiopulmonary criteria, who either suffered cardiac arrest in the hospital or who arrived there dead. With the acceptance of whole-brain criteria of death, organ procurement shifted to heart-beating cadaveric donors—those persons who were found to be brain-dead while cardiopulmonary functions were mechanically sustained. The shortage of brain-dead heart-beating donors has now refocused attention on the use of non-heart-beating donors (NHBDs).

The use of NHBDs that implicates the dead donor rule involves those cases that are planned or controlled, as opposed to those persons who are brought to the hospital dead. These protocols developed out of family requests to donate organs in situations in which it was unlikely that death would be pronounced on brain death grounds, thus preventing solid organ donation from occurring. Organ donation is a significant positive experience for those facing the death of a loved one; if these families are to have that positive experience, organ donation would have to occur immediately after death has been declared subsequent to withdrawal of life support—the non-heart-beating donor situation.

In controlled NHBD cases a family requests that treatment be withdrawn from a loved one who is terminally ill but not brain dead and that his or her organs then be donated for transplant. To minimize warm ischemic time damaging to organs, ventilatory assistance to the patient may be withdrawn in the operating room, where the family may choose to be present. After withdrawal of life support, the patient's attending physician, who is not part of the organ recovery team, determines whether the heart and respiration have stopped. The physician will then pronounce the patient dead or, to provide an additional margin of safety, in some cases will wait an additional two to five minutes after cardiac function has stopped before pronouncing death. At this point the physician and any family that is present would withdraw, and the transplant team, which has been prepped and waiting in an adjoining room, will enter and retrieve organs from the recently dead cadaver. Studies have shown that organs retrieved in this way suffer little damage and are viable for transplant. . . .

Ethical and legal controversy surrounds the use of controlled NHBDs because of the fear that retrieval of organs in the controlled setting could violate the dead donor rule, in either of two ways. One was that the drugs administered prior to death in NHBD protocols—anticoagulants (heparin) and vasodilators (regitine) to minimize the effects of warm ischemia on organ viability—could hasten or even cause death. . . .

Transplant physicians with experience with these drugs deny that they are administered to hasten death or that they are given in such doses that they could have that effect, and the IOM [Institute of Medicine] found that administering heparin and regitine prior to death to preserve organs generally does not harm the donor and is justifiable as part of routine preparation for organ retrieval. . . . Careful attention to whether such drugs need to be administered to the near-death patient to preserve organs and whether the dosages used are contraindicated because of the patient's condition should minimize the risk that efforts to preserve organs prior to death will inadvertently violate the dead donor rule.

> *The dead donor rule plays an important role in protecting persons and engendering trust in a voluntary system of organ donation.*

A second way in which NHBD protocols are said to violate the dead donor rule is that they allow retrieval of organs before cessation of pulmonary function is irreversible. The risk is that death will be pronounced so quickly after the removal of life support and induction of cardiac arrest that the person will not have irreversibly lost cardiac function and thus will still be alive when organs are removed. That is, the person will appear to be dead, but might actually, if given longer time to breathe on his own or if immediately resuscitated, regain spontaneous respiration and circulation. If organ retrieval has already begun in such patients, retrieval will then be the cause of death, thus violating the dead donor rule.

To guard against such mistakes, NHBD programs have traditionally waited a few minutes after determining that cardiopulmonary function has ceased before pronouncing death and beginning organ retrieval. . . .

The debate over the use of NHBDs shows that their use in accordance with guidelines such as those recommended by the IOM does comply with the dead donor rule. Unlike the case of anencephaly, where the donor is clearly alive under whole-brain criteria of death when vital organs are taken, the use of NHBDs involves: no violation of the dead donor rule and requires no public alteration or exception to it. Nevertheless, it is important that NHBDs are used only according to publicly announced protocols that contain clear procedures for minimizing the risk of any such violations. Such protocols should require that death is pronounced according to the attending physician's judgment without pressure from transplant personnel, that tests and waiting periods are used that are reasonably certain to correctly ascertain cardiopulmonary death, and that administration of anticoagulants or vasodilators does not occur in circumstances that might hasten death or harm patients.

Change and the dead donor rule

The dead donor rule plays an important role in protecting persons and engendering trust in a voluntary system of organ donation. Any change in the rule to increase organ supply requires convincing evidence that more benefit than harm to persons and the transplant system would result from such a change. Even then, strong resistance to modifying the rule would exist based on the prudential and symbolic advantages of strict maintenance of a rule against death by organ retrieval.

It is thus no surprise that none of the proposals for explicit exceptions to the dead donor rule have been adopted. Removing vital organs from anencephalic infants requires public recognition that such lives are so diminished or lacking in value that they may be killed for their organs. Although these newborns will imminently die and will suffer no harm from retrieval of vital organs, the symbolic costs of relaxing the dead donor rule appear to be too great to be tolerated. Similarly, organ retrieval executions have little support, despite their attempt to wring some good from society's deliberate taking of life.

The use of NHBDs, on the other hand, is morally and legally acceptable because of their careful attempt to respect the dead donor rule. The debate over the use of NHBDs, however, illustrates the strong opposition that probably would exist if vital organs were taken from non-heart-beating donors who were not dead or if drugs administered to preserve organs also caused death. Despite the briefness and poor quality of the life remaining to such donors, violation of the dead donor rule would most likely be as strongly opposed here as it is with anencephalic infants.

The conservative posture that now exists toward maintaining the dead donor rule is likely to continue for some time, but not because of logical necessity. One could imagine that the question of how strictly the dead donor rule should be adhered to in order to maintain respect for persons and trust in the organ procurement system might be answered differently as medical, ethical, and social conditions and perceptions change. We might, for example, come to accept that persons who have only brain stem function or who are permanently unconscious are so close to being dead that we are willing to take their vital organs when clear benefits to others could be shown. Opponents or proponents of capital punishment might come to accept the need to save lives even as executions occur, and support execution by organ retrieval. Only a slight shift in attitude would then be needed to view the transplant team's role in executions as life-affirming, just as it is in organ retrievals from brain-dead, heart-beating cadavers whose cardiopulmonary functions are ended by organ retrieval. Such shifts in the strictness of the dead donor rule could occur without impairing respect for human life generally or diluting perceptions of physicians as healers, because the life at stake in these cases is so marginal in quality or expectancy and the resulting preservation of life in recipients is so significant.

Yet it is highly unlikely that such changes in perception or practice will soon occur. The symbolic importance of the dead donor rule is so great that even the slightest explicit deviation from it confronts a very high presumption of unacceptability. An important factor in strictly maintaining the rule is the small number of lives that would be saved as a result. With roughly fifty executions and fifty anencephalic births occurring each year, and only a portion of these prisoners or families likely to opt for organ donation, relatively few lives would be saved at the price of crossing an important symbolic threshold. Of course, any additional contribution to the pool of donor organs is welcome. Each cadaveric donor made possible by changes in the dead donor rule could save or extend the lives of three or more existing individuals. But saving the lives of others, as the dead donor rule itself shows, has never been a uniformly privileged activity. Efforts to increase organ supply would be more fruitfully directed to increasing acceptance of NHBDs and the desirability of donating organs generally than to changing the dead donor rule.

11

Advances in Tissue Engineering Could Alleviate the Organ Shortage

Doug Garr

Doug Garr is a business writer, reporter, author, biographer, and corporate communications specialist.

Advances in a field known as tissue engineering could make replacement bladders and blood vessels a reality in the near future, while grown-in-the-lab hearts, lungs, and livers are a longer-term goal. Tissue engineering combines biotechnology procedures, computer technology, the use of microscopic polymers, and other techniques to literally grow organs in the laboratory. The hope is that organs might one day be grown from a patient's own cells, thus reducing or eliminating the chance that a patient's body will reject the transplant.

It's a decade from now, and an elderly man gets the grim news that his heart is rapidly decaying and that the left ventricle—the chamber that squeezes blood out to the body—needs to be replaced. His physician takes a biopsy of the heart cells that are still healthy and ships the tissue to a lab that is really an organ factory. There, workers use the patient's own cells and special polymers to fashion and grow a replacement part—certified by the original manufacturer. In three months, the new ventricle is frozen, packaged and sent to the hospital, where the patient undergoes a standard surgical procedure: the insertion of a living implant created from his own tissue. The surgery saves his life.

Not long ago, the notion of designing and growing living replacement body parts—a process now known as tissue engineering—seemed pure fantasy. But researchers in biotechnology are confident that the day will come when scenarios like the one above will be real and commonplace, thanks to advances made in the last decade in "biomaterials" that are compatible with living cells and the cultivation of new tissue, and to a far better understanding of how cells actually behave. The only question

From "The Human Body Shop," by Doug Garr, *Technology Review,* April 2001. Copyright © 2001 by The Alumni Association of MIT. Reprinted with permission.

is, when? Some predict that within 20 years, possibly sooner, replacement ventricles, bladders, and the like will be readily available. For complex organs like lungs, though, it could take until mid-century.

A run on organs

For ill patients, breakthroughs in tissue-engineered organs can't come soon enough. The shortage of donor organs is infamous. In 1999 (the most recent year for which complete data are available) there were more than 72,000 people in the United States alone on transplant waiting lists, according to statistics from the United Network for Organ Sharing. By year's end, over 6,100 people had died waiting. Dozens of groups in industry and academia are hoping to prevent those deaths, working on techniques for fashioning new organs out of cells from embryos, cadavers or patients themselves, combined with special biomaterials. Most current work in the commercial realm focuses on tissues, valves and other components of organs. Already, there are a handful of tissue-engineered products on the market—skin, bone, and cartilage implants and patches—the first successes in a young field.

Michael Ehrenreich, president of Techvest, a New York–based investment company that closely follows the biotech sector, feels such achievements are only an indication of what's to come, and he is blunt about where tissue engineering is now. "Skin. Big deal. It's a proof of concept," says Ehrenreich. "At the end of the day, many of us are going to die from some sort of organ failure. That's what's going to drive this market. And nobody's really tackled a vascularized organ yet."

Not long ago, the notion of designing and growing living replacement body parts—a process now known as tissue engineering—seemed pure fantasy.

Ehrenreich has touched on one of the more vexing problems facing tissue engineers: most organs need their own vasculature, or network of blood vessels, to get the nutrients they need to survive and to perform their intended functions. So before researchers can build a full-sized organ, such as a liver, say, or a set of lungs, they must learn to manufacture blood vessels.

Growing blood vessels in the lab

Important progress on that front came two years ago, when MIT biomedical engineers Robert Langer and Laura Niklason (now at Duke University Medical Center) grew entire blood vessels from a few cells collected from pigs. Niklason, who led the effort and did much of the work during a stint in Langer's lab, started by taking small biopsies from the carotid arteries of six-month-old miniature swine. She isolated smooth muscle cells from each tissue sample and used those cells to seed the outer surface of a tubular scaffold built of a biodegradable polymer used in sutures. Next, Niklason cultured each new vessel in its own special growth chamber called a bioreactor. Bioreactors are standard in tissue engineering, but in this case there was a twist.

As Langer explains, "What we did is we set up these little pumps that beat like a heart and hooked them up to the artificial blood vessels." The researchers found that the pulsation encouraged the muscle cells to migrate inward, enveloping microscopic fragments of the polymer, and ultimately made the blood vessels much stronger. After growing the vessels in the pulsing environment for several weeks, they added endothelial cells—the thin, flat cells that line the inside of many tissues, including blood vessels—to their inner surfaces, and grew them for a few more days.

Before researchers can build a full-sized organ, such as a liver, say, or a set of lungs, they must learn to manufacture blood vessels.

"That single change totally changed everything," says Langer. "We were actually able to make blood vessels that looked like real vessels." They functioned like real blood vessels too, staying open and clot-free for several weeks when the researchers grafted them into large arteries in the pigs' legs. "The key to getting this to work was to mimic what the body did" by growing the vessels in an environment that pulsed just as a real circulatory system does, says Langer.

While new, artery-sized blood vessels could be a godsend for surgeries like heart bypass, building more complex organs will also require the smallest of blood vessels: capillaries. And since that means tissue engineering on the scale of microns, or millionths of a meter, it's an even greater challenge. To meet that challenge, pediatric surgeon and prominent tissue engineer Joseph Vacanti of Massachusetts General Hospital enlisted the help of colleagues at Draper Laboratory in Cambridge, MA. Vacanti was convinced that the techniques used to etch computer chips could also help build capillaries.

Physicist Jeff Borenstein, who directs Draper's microfabrication program, was encouraged to learn that the smallest human capillary was 10 microns in diameter; he was accustomed to working with computer-chip features about 10 times smaller. "We can draw that with a dull pencil," Borenstein says. "A capillary is like falling off a log for us." The team etched interconnected networks of capillary-like grooves into palm-sized wafers of silicon or Pyrex. In initial experiments, they seeded the wafers with endothelial cells from a rat. The cells grew to line the etched grooves; two cell layers grown this way and sandwiched together formed new vessels that could carry fluid.

In ongoing work, the researchers are instead using the etched wafers as molds in which they cast a biodegradable polymer. The polymer casts can be pulled out of the molds and sandwiched together to form a scaffold for full three-dimensional vessels; then the scaffold can be seeded with endothelial cells. Of course, just one cast's worth of capillaries would not be enough to supply blood to an entire organ. Borenstein once calculated the area of capillary networks needed to support a liver. "It's a pretty large area," he says. "It was something like a small conference-room table for a rat, and a quarter of a football field for an adult human. You can't come up with wafers that are [30 meters] in diameter." So by combining thousands of layers of capillary networks together with liver cells, the researchers hope to create the basic structure for an artificial liver.

Beagle bladders and human hearts

Even without the technology to build extensive vascular systems, one tissue-engineered organ has made it almost all the way to human trials: the bladder. Anthony Atala, a urologist and director of tissue engineering at Children's Hospital, Boston, decided to try to build a bladder in part because it seemed like the easiest organ to begin with. In landmark work done in the late 1990s, Atala's team built new bladders for six beagles. The researchers started by taking a one-centimeter-square biopsy from each dog's natural bladder, isolating the lining cells and the muscle cells from the biopsy, and culturing each cell type separately.

One tissue-engineered organ has made it almost all the way to human trials: the bladder.

After a month, Atala's team had grown enough cells—300 million of each type—to construct an artificial bladder. They used the muscle cells to sheathe the outside of a bladder-shaped polymer scaffold, and the lining cells to cover the inside. The researchers implanted each new bladder into a dog after removing the dog's own bladder. The researchers discovered that not only did blood vessels from the surrounding tissue grow into the tissue-engineered bladder and keep its tissues healthy, but the dogs also had almost as much bladder capacity as dogs with original equipment.

The early work went so well that Atala and Cambridge, MA–based Curis hope to begin the first tests of the new bladder in humans sometime this year. Still, Atala is realistic about what he's already accomplished. For one thing, he has not yet answered the question of how long a bioengineered bladder will last. "With the bladder, it's going to be several years until we know what the long-term results will be," he explains. "We certainly have a good history with skin. Twenty years down the road we know it's fine. With cartilage in the knee, we have a four- or five-year history from the time it was first placed in patients." But with the bladder, Atala says, "We just don't know."

In the meanwhile, Atala's lab has begun to tackle the kidney and has already built small kidney-like units capable of producing urine. Still, given that the kidney is a highly complex structure that includes as many as 20 different types of cells, researchers have to clear many technical hurdles before making full-sized organs for the nearly 48,000 people waiting on kidney transplant lists in the United States alone.

Tissue-engineering a heart will also be a formidable task, but there are a couple of reasons to believe concrete steps in that direction will be made in the not-too-distant future. For one thing, the heart comprises fewer than 10 different cell types. Perhaps even more important, there are two large research consortia targeting the organ. One is the LIFE initiative (for

"Living Implants from Engineering"), begun in 1998 and coordinated by the University of Toronto's Michael Sefton, with the help of a steering committee that includes Massachusetts General Hospital's Vacanti and MIT's Langer. The initiative has marshaled 60 academic and government researchers from North America, Europe and Japan to work on the body's critical pump. Says Sefton, "If we can solve the heart, then the other organs will follow."

Sefton readily admits that a project as enormous as building the heart is, on the face of it, ridiculous. Still, he believes that by breaking the job down into component tasks—isolating human cardiac muscle cells, say, or building flexible scaffolds to support those cells—a consortium of researchers will be able to make it happen.

That model is also being tested, Sefton says, in a university/industry collaboration led by the University of Washington. Financed by a $10 million grant from the National Institutes of Health and including more than 40 researchers, the University of Washington project has broken its undertaking into a series of goals. The first is to generate a tissue-engineered patch that can be grafted onto a damaged heart. Longer term, the researchers hope to build implantable left ventricles, a goal Sefton sees as a "minimoonshot" that could be achieved within the decade. But a fully functional bio-engineered heart, Sefton says, will likely cost billions of dollars—and neither the LIFE initiative nor the University of Washington's has raised that kind of money yet.

Straight from the factory

Ultimately, any method for building new human organs will have to win approval from the U.S. Food and Drug Administration. And that means organ builders will need a standardized, reproducible manufacturing process, says MIT bioengineer Linda Griffith. To achieve that goal, Griffith and her colleagues have turned to a device invented by MIT engineer Emanuel Sachs and used for rapid prototyping and the manufacture of a variety of parts and tools: a three-dimensional powder printer, or 3DP machine.

The first [goal in bio-engineering the human heart] is to generate a tissue-engineered patch that can be grafted onto a damaged heart.

The machine builds up complex shapes layer by layer, based on a computer file capable of depicting the object as a series of horizontal slices. A roller pushes a thin layer of powder across a flat base plate resting on top of a piston. Next, an inkjet printer head distributes a glue, or binder, to solidify the powder only where the blueprint for that slice calls for solid material. The piston then ratchets the plate down by the thickness of the layer, and the process begins again. When all the layers have been printed, the new object can be removed from the machine, and the excess powder falls away.

By adapting the printer to use polymer powders, multiple print heads and special binders, Griffith and her collaborators created a tool capable of mass-producing polymer scaffolds for new tissues and organs. Not only does the printer allow the researchers to control a scaffold's shape with great precision, it also allows them to build in chemical modifications to the structure's surface that help tell different types of cells exactly where and how they should grow.

It's just that sort of fine control that may help tissue engineers conquer even the most complicated organs. Indeed, Griffith is now—along with Vacanti and Princeton, NJ–based Therics—working out ways to manufacture livers and other organs with three-dimensional printing. Griffith already knows a great deal about growing liver tissue; she worked on the details while leading an effort to develop a liver-cell-based biological-weapon detector for the U.S. Defense Advanced Research Projects Agency. The hope is that scientific knowledge, combined with three-dimensional-printing technology, will make building a liver for implantation possible.

If everything pans out as Griffith, Vacanti and their colleagues hope, manufacturing machines could someday hum in FDA-certified organ factories. It's too soon to know if those factories will churn out entire organs on site, or if they'll instead produce and ship elaborate scaffold structures on which doctors will grow patients' own cells, right in the hospital. But either approach, if successful, promises one thing: an end to transplant waiting lists.

12
Animal-to-Human Transplants Could Alleviate the Organ Shortage

Erika Jonietz

Erika Jonietz is an associate editor of Technology Review.

Researchers have been working on animal-to-human organ transplants—called xenotransplantation—since before 1984, when "Baby Fae" received a heart transplant from a baby baboon. Scientists now believe that pigs may be the most suitable animal organ donors, because of their similarity to humans in terms of both biology and size. Many problems must be overcome before pig-to-human transplants become as routine as human-to-human transplants, but the promise of saving some of the thousands who die each year for lack of human organ donors is enough to keep researchers trying.

The numbers are grim. According to the United Network for Organ Sharing, more than three times as many people in the United States were waiting for heart, kidney and liver transplants than received them in 1999; over 5,500 people died waiting for organs. And many more patients could benefit from organ transplants than ever make the waiting list, either because they are too sick or too healthy to qualify. According to one estimate, 45,000 Americans could benefit each year from heart transplants, but only 2,000 or so human hearts are available.

One promising solution to this medical predicament is to harvest organs from suitable animals and use them for human transplant. It may sound outlandish, but several biotech and pharmaceutical heavyweights, as well as some smaller biotech firms, are gearing up to do just that. In preliminary experiments, these companies have already implanted animal cells in human volunteers to treat such diseases as Parkinson's and epilepsy. Researchers plan to start whole-organ clinical trials in the next two to three years.

The use of animal organs in human transplants is not exactly new.

From "A Donor Named Wilbur," by Erika Jonietz, *Technology Review*, May 2001. Copyright © 2001 by The Alumni Association of MIT. Reprinted with permission.

You may remember "Baby Fae," the 12-day-old California infant who, in 1984, received a heart transplant from a most unusual donor—a baby baboon. This controversial experiment marked the first time most people had ever heard of "xeno-transplantation," transplanting tissues or organs between species, and Baby Fae's very public death only 20 days after her surgery chilled the climate for xeno-transplantation work. Still, medical researchers quietly pressed ahead, and their efforts may soon pay off.

The animal of choice in the new generation of experiments? Pigs. That's because pigs are both plentiful and easy to raise, and "the similarities to man are amazing," says Julia Greenstein, CEO of Immerge Bio-Therapeutics, a joint venture between Swiss drug giant Novartis and Charlestown, MA–based BioTransplant.

The animal of choice in the new generation of experiments? Pigs.

But transplanting tissues from pigs to people does present a few problems. The most critical is "hyperacute rejection," an immune reaction that causes organs from pigs to turn black and cease functioning within minutes of transplant into humans. The cause of this reaction is a sugar called alpha-gal that laces the surface of every pig cell. Since human cells don't make this sugar, the immune system produces antibodies against it and kills all cells bearing it.

For whole-organ transplants to become reality, a strategy is needed to deal with the troublesome sugar. That's why companies such as Princeton, NJ–based Nextran are genetically engineering pigs to make proteins that help repress the immune reaction that the sugar causes. Nextran, owned by pharmaceutical giant Baxter, has already used the livers of such pigs to keep patients with acute liver failure alive until donor organs were found. In these early human tests, the pig livers remained outside the body, but "it's just a prelude to going into a human," says University of Pittsburgh transplant surgeon John Fung. The company plans to apply for permission to conduct preliminary human trials of such xenotransplants by the end of next year.

Other companies, including Immerge, PPL Therapeutics and Advanced Cell Technology, are combining this strategy with efforts to completely eliminate the guilty pig sugar. To do this, they must "knock out"—disable or remove entirely—the gene for the enzyme that makes the sugar. There is some concern, however, over whether pigs can survive without the sugar. "Chances are the pigs will be healthy, but no one's 100 percent sure," says immunologist David Cooper of Massachusetts General Hospital's Transplantation Biology Research Center.

Even if the pigs do survive, genetic modifications alone might not be enough to conquer transplant rejection problems, even with antirejection drugs. So PPL, Immerge and Advanced Cell Technology are pursuing additional strategies for blocking rejection. Each hopes to fool the human immune system into thinking that a new pig organ belongs in the body, usually by infusing or implanting pig bone-marrow cells into the recipient several weeks before a transplant operation. The idea is to use antirejection drugs to keep the marrow cells alive long enough for the human immune system to start thinking of the pig cells as "self"—reducing the patient's dependence on very large doses of the powerful drugs after the organ transplant. Fung is skeptical, though: "Trying to get animal organs to be accepted using approaches that haven't worked in human organ transplantation requires a leap of faith."

Research continues

Omaha, NE–based Ximerex is even more ambitious, trying to completely eliminate the need for antirejection drugs by "introducing" individual pigs and transplant recipients prior to surgery. A patient's bone marrow cells would be infused into a pig fetus, educating both the pig and human immune cells to think of each other as self. After the pig's birth, hybrid pig/human bone marrow would be put back into the patient. One drawback: patients would have to wait four to five months between bone marrow sampling and transplant operations. Ximerex president William Beschorner doesn't think the obstacle is insurmountable: "The typical wait for a human transplant is well over a year. It would not be a major problem for most patients."

Each of these companies hopes to begin clinical testing of heart and kidney xenotransplants in the next few years. Although Cooper is generally optimistic, he sounds a note of caution. "It's like peeling an onion: every time you pull off one layer, you find another problem underneath." The thousands who die each year waiting for new organs hope those problems are solved soon.

13
Artificial Organs Could Obviate Many of the Ethical Dilemmas Surrounding Organ Transplants

Economist

The Economist *is a weekly magazine of business and politics.*

The chronic shortage of organs for transplant has led scientists to pursue ethically problematic research, including experiments on cloning human cells and attempting animal-to-human transplants. The need for these controversial techniques could be obviated by the development of artificial organs. Many companies are working to perfect synthetic blood, which promises to alleviate blood donor shortages and the problem of donated blood being tainted with disease and HIV infection. Artificial heart technology is becoming increasingly sophisticated, and artificial livers are in the works. Some companies are also experimenting with artificial lungs, bones, and skin.

Where once they seemed utopian, early promises by genetic engineers to stave off disease, replenish stocks of organs and rejuvenate populations now appear unacceptable, even intimidating. To work these miracles of modern medicine, biologists need to explore genetic modification, stem-cell research and xenotransplantation (use of animal organs in humans). But the public outcry against such research has resulted in most of it being heavily regulated or banned outright.

Making matters worse, these research tools have proved difficult to use in therapy. Even one of the least controversial, but most valuable, applications of such research—growing healthy adult organs from adult stem cells—now seems decades off. Without such technology, the shortage of donor organs and the growing toll of diabetes and heart disease will only get worse.

The good news is that a number of companies are seeking remedies

From "The New Organ-Grinders," *Economist*, June 23, 2001. Copyright © 2001 by Economist Newspapers Ltd. Reprinted with permission.

for such afflictions that avoid the political and scientific challenges posed by cloning. They are developing substitute blood and guts using traditional engineering metals, chemicals and plastics held together with nuts and bolts. Within a couple of years, repairing patients could be more like fixing worn out motor cars.

Within a couple of years, repairing patients could be more like fixing worn out motor cars.

According to the World Health Organisation, heart disease is the deadliest ailment in the world. Thousands of patients need new hearts annually; most die waiting. In the next 25 years, as the number of diabetics worldwide doubles to 300m, the demand for fake pancreases will soar. Add to that an ageing population that is going to need better hearing, eyesight and livers. No surprise that the bionics industry is enjoying such robust growth.

Artificial blood

One of the most eagerly-awaited products is artificial blood. Getting people to donate blood of different types in sufficient quantities is costly and time-consuming for clinics. Much of it goes to waste. After six weeks, stored blood starts to spoil and must be discarded. Collection clinics must certify each donation to be free of diseases such as HIV and hepatitis. But as recent tragedies have shown, such tests are far from foolproof. When labour costs are included, the price of a typical 250-millilitre unit of blood is $200–250. A proposal to filter out white blood cells, which may irritate some patients, could raise the price by a further $30–40.

Companies that make artificial blood are eager to cater for this demand, which amounts to some 14m units a year in America alone. The market for artificial blood in the United States is supplied by a Canadian firm called Hemosol and three American companies, Biopure, Northfield Laboratories and Alliance Pharmaceuticals. Hemosol, Biopure and Northfield manufacture solutions of purified haemoglobin, the molecule in blood that transports oxygen throughout the body. The Hemosol and Northfield products use haemoglobin that is harvested from human blood, while Biopure uses haemoglobin purified from cows. Such products are a sort of "eau de blood", providing haemoglobin's oxygen-carrying capacity without any of its infectious or abrasive ingredients.

Alliance's product, called Oxygene, takes this a step further. Oxygene contains no animal or human blood products whatsoever, being a milky emulsion of salt water and a compound called perflubron. The attraction of perflubron is that its molecules stow oxygen in their core. When they float past oxygen-starved tissue, the perflubron molecules swap their oxygen for carbon dioxide more readily than does human haemoglobin. After a day or so in the bloodstream, the perflubron evaporates and is exhaled harmlessly by the patient. All of these blood substitutes are disease-free, cost about the same as natural blood, and have a shelf life of one to three years.

The best thing about artificial blood is that, containing no nasty proteins, it works with all blood types. Man-made organs are similarly compatible. Some get their universal appeal from the innocuous materials out of which they are made. Others make themselves acceptable by hiding their potential threats from the body's immune system. This special attribute of artificial organs in general—universal compatibility—is what has kick-started the business and attracted the hot money.

Not without reason. More than 75,000 Americans are waiting for a suitable organ to be donated. Only one in three will be lucky enough to get a transplant. And those that do will have to remain on a harsh regimen of drugs for the rest of their lives—to prevent their immune systems from rejecting the foreign tissue.

Artificial hearts

The idea of a totally artificial heart has set medical pulses racing. The first working attempt to make such a device, Jarvik-7, was tried out in several patients during the early 1980s. The problem with Jarvik-7 was that it required patients to remain constantly tethered to a machine the size of a refrigerator. Worse still, it caused deaths from clots and infection. Since then, artificial hearts have been used only as "bridges to transplant"—to tide patients over while a donor heart was found.

That has begun to change. Several American and Canadian firms are now getting regulatory approval for artificial heart devices that will remain in the body permanently. One device called AbioCor, which is made by Abiomed of Danvers, Massachusetts, replaces the natural heart entirely. Others, such as the HeartSaver from World Heart of Ottawa, replace or augment only the activity of the left ventricle—the lower chamber that pumps the blood through the body. Since it is the left ventricle that collapses in most cases of heart failure, such a "left-ventricular assist device" often provides enough help to allow the heart to start beating again with much of its natural tissue intact.

The best thing about artificial blood is that, containing no nasty proteins, it works with all blood types. Man-made organs are similarly compatible.

Made from materials such as titanium and Dacron, artificial hearts use a sensor to gauge the blood flow and a chamber to hold the blood while it is pumped by a battery-powered rotor. Oddly, a pulse is optional. Both the AbioCor and the HeartSaver generate one to keep the patient happy. The device rests in the chest cavity adjacent to the real heart. The internal batteries that power the device are recharged through the skin without the need for wires. A magnetic coil laid against the abdomen induces an electrical current in a matching magnetic coil stowed inside the patient's body.

Both Abiomed and World Heart have incorporated additional sensors to monitor such vital signs as heart rate and blood pressure. The HeartSaver will be able to transmit such data to a local controller using an infrared wireless signal. With the control unit linked to the Internet, hospitals will be able continuously to monitor patients fitted with artificial hearts. Better still, a doctor in a hospital who notices that the device is beating too slowly could send instructions over the Internet to tell it to speed up.

Every part of the human body is now being studied to see how it can be replicated artificially or augmented in some way.

World Heart already has approval for long-term use of its HeartSaver in Europe. The company hopes to start human trials in Canada before the end of the year. And now that the FDA has approved clinical trials in America, the first AbioCor could be implanted in a human patient by June. Initially, such a mechanical heart would cost as much as $60,000–100,000, though the price could fall by half once the device goes into mass production. Even after adding a further $40,000 for surgery, the total bill for installing an artificial heart would be considerably less than the $200,000 that transplanting a donor heart costs today.

Despite its ingenuity, the mechanics of the natural heart are relatively straightforward. Even severed from nerves, it will continue to beat when placed in a bucket of correctly salted water. By contrast, other organs of the body are more multifunctional. And simulating them requires more complicated equipment.

Artificial pancreases and livers

Take the pancreas. This senses levels of glucose in the blood and releases insulin accordingly. MiniMed, a firm based in Northridge, California, manufactures external insulin pumps that can be programmed by patients to deliver appropriate doses of insulin. It is also testing a sensor that can continuously monitor blood sugar levels. Once the company mates these two technologies, the external pump could automatically gauge and administer microdoses of insulin. MiniMed hopes to make an implantable pump-and-sensor, thus erasing all evidence of the disease and its cure.

But designing and building such sensors and chemical pumps is costly. One alternative is to use nature's own equivalents—ie, living cells. Circe Biomedical of Lexington, Massachusetts, is testing an implantable "bio-artificial" pancreas that contains living pancreatic cells taken from pigs. The patient's blood flows through a graft into a membraneous tube that is surrounded by the pig pancreatic tissue. Through the membrane, the cells detect the level of glucose in the human bloodstream and release insulin as required. But since the pig cells are encased in a plastic housing, the patient's immune system never detects their presence—and therefore never mounts an attack. Every few months, the supply of pig pancreas cells is washed out and replenished through portholes that are embedded in the patient's abdomen.

Circe and other firms are pursuing a similar approach with artificial livers. No mechanical device has yet come close to replicating the host of chemical actions performed by liver cells. They cleanse the blood, break down and build complex molecules, and keep the blood volume on an even keel. So the artificial livers in development use actual liver cells—from pigs as well as from people—to do their chemical work for them. Such machines could be used to support patients in critical condition while they wait for a liver to be found for transplant.

Artificial livers work in much the same way as do kidney-dialysis machines. Blood is taken from the body, cleaned, treated and then replaced. As blood is collected from the patient's body, the fluid portion ("plasma") is extracted and the blood cells and other solid matter set aside. The plasma is then pushed through a charcoal column to extract the toxic chemicals. Next, it is oxygenated so that it can do its basic job and then enters a so-called bioreactor.

The bioreactor contains up to 5,000 hollow tubes made of a flexible membrane, clustered together in a plastic cylinder. Liver cells that have been cultured to grow on the outer surface of these tubes freely exchange biological molecules and water with blood passing through the membrane. As with the artificial pancreas, the membrane screens the foreign cells from the patient's immune system, which never realises that interlopers are meddling with its blood supply.

VitaGen of La Jolla, California, takes a similar approach, but with an important difference. Instead of pig cells or normal human cells, the firm uses a patented line of cloned human cells that are bred to be immortal. VitaGen's device is being tested in America. Meanwhile, Circe's Hepat-Assist should finish its clinical trials by the end of 2001.

Only the beginning

Such technologies for making artificial organs are only the beginning. Every part of the human body is now being studied to see how it can be replicated artificially or augmented in some way. Biomedical engineers at the University of Pittsburgh Medical Centre are developing prototypes of an artificial lung that can be strapped on a belt, rather like a mobile phone or personal digital assistant. A team led by William Federspiel, a veteran of Abiomed's artificial heart team, is working on an intravenous oxygenator that exchanges gas with the blood as it passes through a set of hollow fibres. A firm called Optobionics, based in Wheaton, Illinois, is trying to create a silicon chip that stimulates the visual cortex and may help to restore sight to the blind. And various types of substitute cartilage, bone and skin are working their way through clinical trials.

The technical hurdles that such firms have already overcome also lay the groundwork for future achievements. Most notably, they extend the range and capabilities of membranes that are safe to put inside the human body. They provide means for inserting power supplies within flesh. They allow animal tissue to be used safely in people. And, best of all, they detach the whole business of organ replacement from the tricky ethical questions associated with genetics, returning the endeavour to the practical, non-controversial realm of chemical and electronic engineering.

Organizations to Contact

The editors have compiled the following list of organizations concerned with the issues debated in this book. The descriptions are derived from materials provided by the organizations. All have publications or information available for interested readers. The list was compiled on the date of publication of the present volume; the information provided here may change. Be aware that many organizations take several weeks or longer to respond to inquiries, so allow as much time as possible.

American Organ Transplant Association (AOTA)
3335 Cartwright Rd., Missouri City, TX 77459
(281) 261-AOTA

The association is a nonprofit organization that works to make transplant surgery available to anyone that needs it. AOTA works with people to help them raise funds for their transplants, directs them to hospitals that perform the type of transplant surgery they require, and contracts with Continental Airlines and Greyhound Lines to provide complimentary airline and bus service to patients and their families who cannot afford to pay for transportation to transplant centers. AOTA's booklet, *Life After Transplantation,* discusses the types of medications all transplant recipients must take for the rest of their lives, as well as the side effects of these medications and ways to cope with them.

American Society of Transplant Surgeons (ASTS)
1020 North Fairfax St., Suite 200, Alexandria, VA 22314
(888) 990-2787
website: www.asts.org

The ASTS consists of surgeons, physicians, and nonphysician scientists who are actively engaged in transplantation. It publishes the *American Journal of Transplantation* and posts statements about ethics and public policy on its website.

Campaign for Responsible Transplantation (CRT)
PO Box 2751, New York, NY 10163-2751
(212) 579-3477
website: www.crt-online.org

The campaign is a nonprofit organization launched in 1998 out of concern over the rush to commercialize animal-to-human organ transplantation (xenotransplantation) using genetically modified pigs and nonhuman primates. CRT believes that xenotransplantation poses a grave danger to human health because of the risk of transferring deadly animal viruses to the human population, and is mounting a petition to ban xenotransplantation research. News updates, press releases, and other resources are available on the CRT website.

Center for Bioethics
University of Pennsylvania
3401 Market St. #320, Philadelphia, PA 19104
(215) 898-3453
website: www.bioethics.net

The Center for Bioethics at the University of Pennsylvania is the largest bioethics center in the world, and it runs the world's first and largest bioethics website. Its members engage in research on and publish many articles about the ethics of organ transplants. *PennBioethics* is its quarterly newsletter.

Hastings Center
Route 9D, Garrison, NY 10524-5555
(914) 424-4040
website: www.hastingscenter.org

The Hastings Center is an independent research institute that explores the medical, ethical, and social ramifications of biomedical advances. The center publishes books, papers, guidelines, and the bimonthly *Hastings Center Report*.

International Society for Heart and Lung Transplantation (ISHLT)
14673 Midway Rd., Suite 200, Addison, TX 75001
(972) 490-9495
website: www.ishlt.org

ISHLT is a not-for-profit organization of doctors and scientists dedicated to the advancement of the science and treatment of end-stage heart and lung diseases. The society publishes a newsletter and the *Journal of Heart and Lung Transplantation.*

Organ Keeper
PO Box 4413, Middletown, RI 02842
website: www.organkeeper.com

Organ Keeper believes the government's organ donation policies have created an organ donor shortage. It promotes market-based alternatives to the current system of procurement and allocating human organs for transplantation.

TransWeb
The Northern Brewery
1327 Jones Dr., Suite 105, Ann Arbor, MI 48105
website: www.transweb.org

TransWeb is a nonprofit educational website serving the world transplant community. Based at the University of Michigan, TransWeb features news and events, real people's experiences, the top ten myths about donation, a donation quiz, and a large collection of questions and answers, as well as a reference area with everything from articles to videos.

Uncaged Campaigns
St. Matthews House
45 Carver St., 2nd Floor, Sheffield S1 4FT, UK
+44 (0) 114 272 2220
website: www.uncaged.co.uk

Uncaged Campaigns is an animal rights organization based in the United Kingdom. Its members oppose animal-to-human transplants on scientific and ethical grounds and promote vegan, feminist, and green philosophies.

United Network for Organ Sharing (UNOS)
PO Box 13770, Richmond, VA 23225
(804) 330-8500
website: www.unos.org

UNOS is a system of transplant and organ procurement centers, tissue-typing labs, and transplant surgical teams. It was formed to help organ donors and people who need organs to find each other. By federal law, organs used for transplants must be cleared through UNOS. The network also formulates and implements national policies on equal access to organs and organ allocation, organ procurement, and AIDS testing. It publishes the monthly *UNOS Update*.

Bibliography

Books

Arthur L. Caplan and Daniel H. Coelho, eds.	*The Ethics of Organ Transplants: The Current Debate.* Amherst, NY: Prometheus Books, 1998.
Robert Finn	*Organ Transplants: Making the Most of Your Gift of Life.* Sebastopol, CA: O'Reilly, 2000.
Austen Garwood-Gowers	*Living Donor Organ Transplantation: Key Legal and Ethical Issues.* Brookfield, VT: Ashgate/Dartmouth, 1999.
E. Richard Gold	*Body Parts: Property Rights and the Ownership of Human Biological Materials.* Washington, DC: Georgetown University Press, 1996.
Andrew Kimbrell	*The Human Body Shop: The Engineering and Marketing of Life.* Washington, DC: Regnery, 1998.
David Lamb	*Organ Transplants and Ethics.* Brookfield, VT: Avebury, 1996.
Margaret Lock	*Twice Dead: Organ Transplants and the Reinvention of Death.* Berkeley: University of California Press, 2002.
David Price	*Legal and Ethical Aspects of Organ Transplantation.* New York: Cambridge University Press, 2000.
Paula Trzepcaz and Andrea F. DiMartini, eds.	*The Transplant Patient: Biological, Psychiatric, and Ethical Issues in Organ Transplantation.* New York: Cambridge University Press, 2000.
Stuart J. Youngner, Renée C. Fox, and Laurence J. O'Connell, eds.	*Organ Transplantation: Meanings and Realities.* Madison: University of Wisconsin Press, 1996.

Periodicals

Helen Buttery	"When Does Life End?: Questions Persist over the 'Brain Death' Concept in Organ Transplants," *Maclean's*, January 28, 2002.
Charles D. Carlstrom and Christy D. Rollow	"Organ Transplant Shortages: A Matter of Life and Death," *USA Today*, November 1999.
Charles D. Carlstrom and Christy D. Rollow	"The Rationing of Organ Transplants: A Troubled Lineup," *Cato Journal*, Fall 1997. Available from the Cato Institute, 1000 Massachusetts Ave. NW, Washington, DC 20001-5403 or www.cato.org.
Avery Comarow	"Transplant to a Friend," *U.S. News & World Report*, July 23, 2001.

Economist	"The Return of the Bodysnatchers: The Organ-Removal Scandal," May 19, 2001.
John Fischman	"How to Build a Body Part," *Time*, March 1, 1999.
Sanjay Gupta	"A Better Way to Give a Heart," *Time*, December 10, 2001.
Harper's	"Habeus Corpus," February 2002.
Issues and Controversies On File	"Organ Allocation," May 16, 1997.
Robert Kunzig	"The Beat Goes On," *Discover*, January 2000.
Life	"Need a New Nose? A New Heart? Someday Doctors May Be Able to Grow You One," October 15, 1998.
Christina S. Melvin and Barbara S. Heater	"Organ Donation: Moral Imperative or Outrage?" *Nursing Forum*, October–December 2001.
Steven Nadis	"We Can Rebuild You," *Technology Review*, October 1997.
Dorothy Nelkin and Lori Andrews	"*Homo Economicus*: Commercialization of Body Tissue in the Age of Biotechnology," *Hastings Center Report*, September/October 1998.
Newsweek	"A Pig Could Someday Save Your Life," January 1, 2000.
Robert Pool	"Saviors," *Discover*, May 1998.
David J. Rothman	"The International Organ Traffic," *New York Times Review of Books*, March 26, 1998.
Ziauddin Sardar	"Animal Magic," *New Statesman*, November 27, 1998.
Craig S. Smith	"Quandary in U.S. over Use of Organs of Chinese Inmates," *New York Times*, November 11, 2001.
Sheryl Stolberg	"Pennsylvania Set to Break the Taboo on Reward for Organ Donations," *New York Times*, May 6, 1999.
Karen Wright	"The Body Bazaar," *Discover*, October 1998.

Index